THE OBESE BRAIN

How the brain holds the key in the battle against obesity

L. Jiménez

© 2014 Luis Jiménez, first Spanish version

© 2016 Paul Trollope, English translation

First English edition: May 2016

ISBN: 978-1533323538

Dedicated to my mother, who will always be there.

CONTENT

Introduction   7

PART 1 – THE BRAIN, APPETITE AND SATIETY   13

1.1. The central super-super processing unit   15

1.2. The energy regulator   29

1.3. Eating gives us pleasure   45

PART 2 – A MALADJUSTED BRAIN   67

2.1. When the "thermostat" goes wrong   71

2.2. Emotions and addictions   103

2.3. A duped brain   137

PART 3 – REPROGRAMMING THE BRAIN   157

3.1. Fixing the "thermostat"   159

3.2. Treating an addiction   179

3.3. A motivated brain   195

3.4. For the powers that be   223

INTRODUCTION

The mere fact that you're reading this probably means you have a particular interest in food and its relation with health. It's also possible you may be overweight. In either case, I'm going to assume that you're a reasonably well informed person who does not need me to remind you of the current epidemic of obesity in our society and the importance of nutrition for people's wellbeing. In fact, you've no doubt read numerous publications on these subjects and are already well aware of the fact that, if there's one thing all developed countries have in common, it's that the weight of their citizens is spiralling upwards.

This book deals with those issues of obesity, food and health. It's not the first book I've written: in my two previous books, "What science tells us about losing weight" and "What science tells us about diets, nutrition and health", I address these issues from a dietary perspective based on epidemiological studies and clinical trials. Those first two books were designed to generally raise readers' awareness of what science knows (and doesn't know) about nutrition and health, pointing out existing misinformation on the subject and explaining the most recommended eating patterns, all with a view to providing the reader with a reasonably solid base on which to take their own personal decisions. However, both those books address the issue mainly from the perspective of eating habits, as I believed, based on scientific evidence, that an individual's regular diet is one of the main factors, if not the most important factor, in weight gain with no apparent solution.

This book reframes the issue from a different perspective: not because the essence of the problem has changed (I don't think it has) and neither because what we eat is no longer a key factor (I'm convinced that it is), but because one of the most intriguing aspects of the whole issue for me is that which analyses the subject from the perspective of our brain. This approach looks at the issues of behaviour and metabolism on an integrated basis but in a slightly different way, using the disciplines of neurobiology, psychiatry and psychology: in other words, through "mind-coloured glasses".

In short, the aim of this book is to provide answers to the following questions:

Why do we eat when we eat?

What drives us to eat too much?

What can we do to avoid this?

All of which, from a cerebral perspective, can be summed up in one question:

Why does our brain sometimes make us eat too much?

The answers to these questions will necessarily be revealed step by step, stage by stage. Firstly, we'll look at how our brain, that incredible machine behind everything we do and the central character throughout this book, works, and later, we'll look at the close relationship between this organ and food, since the brain houses the nucleus which manages the desire to eat.

In the field of diet therapy, the most reliable and rigorous studies and trials on food and health are all relatively recent, thereby giving us no option other than to wait a little longer for solid and comprehensive scientific support to enable us to understand and combat obesity. This scenario is even more precarious in the case of the neurological and psychological perspective, as science is at a considerably more fledgling stage in these specialities. Furthermore, and for obvious reasons, the studies required are more complex to conduct: for example, the amount of food eaten and energy consumed can be monitored and controlled quite precisely in a clinical trial on foodstuffs, but to define, measure and assess a certain behaviour, feeling, sensation or mental reaction presents a rather more complicated challenge. In any case, the amount of research work is increasing exponentially and, as an appetiser of what the future may reveal, I believe that some exciting conclusions and interesting hypotheses on the subject can already be drawn on the basis of the results currently available to us.

The structure and layout of this book will be similar to that of the previous ones. Reference will be made (at the end of each section, so as not to get in the reader's way while reading) to publications, books and scientific studies conducted to date on each subject. In this sense, and particularly for the sake of those readers who have not read my previous books and are not familiar with the studies involved, I would like to very briefly explain the three general types of research which exist.

The most common type of research is what we'll call "observational study", in the course of which large quantities of information (on weight, illnesses, diet, habits, cholesterol, blood pressure, life expectancy, etc.) are compiled on a large sample group of people over a given and specific period of time. A statistical analysis is subsequently made of the associations between each of the variables, with a view to identifying possible correlations (for example, an increase in cholesterol is associated with increased mortality). The major drawback with this type of study is that it is practically impossible to isolate direct correlations between two specific variables (in the previous example, cholesterol and mortality) and derive a cause-effect relation (cholesterol increases mortality), as there are often other variables which are not possible to properly isolate (people with higher cholesterol levels are normally more sedentary, a factor which may increase mortality) and which influence the result.

The second type of study, so-called "clinical trials", can be considered as more rigorous than observational studies and more interesting in terms of drawing clinical conclusions. Clinical trials consist of intervening, or introducing a specific change, in a sample group of people (for example, adding a particular foodstuff, providing medication, including a new habit, etc.) and monitoring the consequences over, and at the end of, a period of time, preferably comparing the findings with those of a control group not subject to the same change. In this case, results may be more reliable for establishing causality conclusions, as something has been introduced artificially and in a relatively isolated manner. Furthermore, comparison is being made with another reference group in which there has been no intervention.

The third type of study is called "reviews". Basically, these reviews compile the results of a series of studies (observational and/or intervention), analyse them, evaluate them, give them weightings and draw corresponding conclusions. For obvious reasons, a review of intervention studies will normally produce more reliable results than a review of observational studies. The type of review considered to be the most rigorous is the meta-analysis, in which a highly structured methodology is followed at all stages. Both quantitative and qualitative valuations are drawn from the results of these studies.

For those of you not familiar with the vagaries of scientific literature, it may seem rather strange that different studies may come up with contradictory results. This is normal in disciplines, such as medicine, which are not an exact science. No two people are the same, and the variables which may affect those people and the processes of the trial are multiple. Many coinciding studies are therefore required to reach conclusions which may be safely extrapolated as general findings. For this very reason, excessive value should not be given to the findings from any one individual study.

I would also like to clarify that I have chosen the references cited at the end of each section on the basis of two criteria: firstly, to back up the statements made in the text, for you to check that the hypotheses presented are substantiated, that what I'm putting forward are proposals and approaches developed by scientists and experts in their respective fields and not something I have simply pulled out of thin air; and secondly, to provide complementary information for those of you interested in further reading on one or other of these issues. I have, therefore, sought out a considerable number of open access publications for those of you with no access to commercial scientific journals (for which there is normally a fee). If you would like to consult one or another of the studies, simply type the title of the study into a search engine such as Google and it will appear on your screen in a matter of seconds.

So, I won't keep you any longer, aware that you're probably keen to find out more about what this new perspective on obesity has to offer. I'll just tell you in advance that, as the title of the book suggests, it's highly likely that the key to the battle against obesity lies therein.

At least, that's what science is telling us.

PART 1

THE BRAIN, APPETITE AND SATIETY

1.1. THE CENTRAL SUPER-SUPERPROCESSING UNIT

The brain, that wrinkly walnut-shaped organ that takes up most of the space in your head and which at times can require up to a quarter of all the energy your body has to consume, is the core of your central nervous system. In engineering terms, it could be seen as the general control unit, the equivalent of a central microprocessor in a computer. The function of the brain is to control the activity of all the other organs of the body using the huge amount of information constantly channelled through to it, for example, by our five senses, and especially through the chemical and physical signals generated as a result of the myriad metabolic and biochemical processes continuously occurring in the human body. It also sends out the requisite orders for all those organs to respond appropriately, ensuring they function as a coordinated whole.

But that's not all the story. On an emotional level (we'll be returning to this aspect repeatedly in this book), the brain plays a key role. It's home to the innermost and most intimate "you", what some refer to as your soul and what scientists call consciousness. Strictly speaking, it could be said that your brain is you, or that you are your brain.

The brain is not exclusive to man: evolution has provided practically all animals with a brain. Apart from in the case of a few invertebrates such as sponges, jellyfish and starfish, the brain, that most complex of all existing organs, would seem to be a very effective system for orchestrating the different parts and components of all living creatures of the animal kingdom. Though there are, as we shall see later, important differences between the brain of one species and another, its basic units are always the same. All brains are made up of two large groups of cells: neurons and glial cells. Neurons, more widely known and considered as more important, are interconnected and generate electrical and chemical flows in the brain (we'll look at this later in more detail). On the other hand, glial cells, also referred to as neuroglia or simply glia, not only provide metabolic and structural support for neurons but also, as has recently been discovered, help form the connections between them and participate in different ways. Though we still have a lot to learn about glia, they can be seen as a type of "nutritional concrete" to help hold neurons in place.

However, there are several characteristics of the human brain which distinguish it from those of animals. Not only is the human brain exceptionally large in proportion to body size (the brain size to body mass ratio), the balance of neurons and glia is also different from that in an animal brain. There are an estimated ten times more glia than neurons in the human brain, whilst in less sophisticated brains such as that of a fly, this proportion is reversed.

Another distinguishing feature of the human brain is its unique capacity to grow as we grow. When we are born, our brain is similar in size to that of a chimpanzee. However, as we develop, the human brain grows much more in comparison, especially the cerebral cortex (the outer layer). It is precisely this area of the brain that houses the most advanced brain functions and those most closely related to intelligence. What's more, the period of our lives when the brain increases most dramatically in size is when we learn most new things: our childhood.

The brain in figures

As I've already mentioned, the brain requires exceptional amounts of energy. During infancy, the period of our lives when new connections are being generated most intensively and the brain is developing at its greatest rate, the amount of energy the brain requires has been estimated at up to 40% of the total energy consumption of the body, far in excess of the 20-25% required on a regular basis during adult life. This percentage figure is, any case, far higher than that of any other animal.

This huge need for resources may explain why human infancy lasts so long compared to that of other animals. Some theories suggest that the rest of the body has to "wait its turn" and make do with the energy the brain leaves available for it.

Another unique feature of the human brain is its tremendous complexity. The numbers involved tell their own story: there are over eighty billion neurons in the brain, enabling it to form trillions of synapses (connections). To put these figures into perspective, eighty billion is over ten times more than the total number of people on our planet.

However, the most fascinating characteristic of these very special cells is, without doubt, their interconnectivity and capacity to transmit electrochemical signals through these connections. Furthermore, their remarkable physical appearance shows how perfectly they are adapted to this very specific function. Most (though not all) neurons are equipped at one end with what looks like a profusion of branches or tentacles called dendrites, which are specialised in connecting with other neurons and may appear in very variable and multiple quantities. All dendrites extrude from the soma, or cell body, which contains the nucleus. Additionally, a single, long and thin filament known as the axon also extrudes from the soma. The axon is a type of conductor cable for transmitting signals and may extend for a considerable distance. The axon may connect with the dendrites of another cell.

The structure of a typical neuron is shown below:

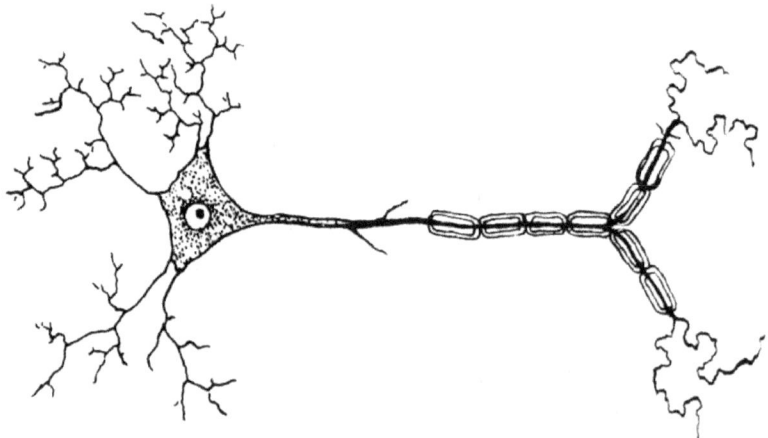

The soma (containing the nucleus) can be seen on the left, surrounded by dendrites. The end of the axon can be seen to the far right.

A cluster of neurons looks something like this:

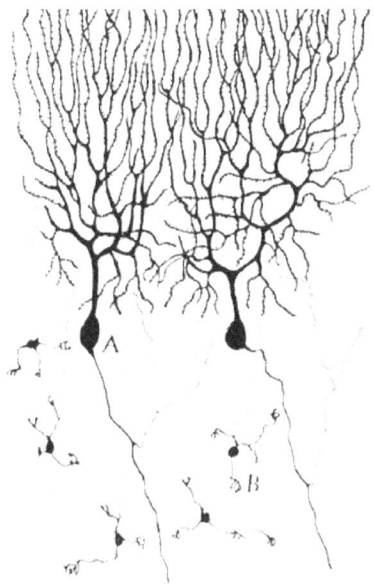

An electrical miracle

One of the most singular and crucial features of neurons is their electrical excitability and sensitivity. An uneven distribution of positive and negative ions produces a difference in electrical charge between the inner and outer cell of a neuron, a fundamental condition for neuronal interconnection through the process known as *synapse*. A synapse between two neurons can be simplified by running through the following sequence of biochemical events:

1. An electrical signal triggers the release through axon terminals of various chemical compounds synthesized from simple precursors such as amino acids (they are, therefore, often proteins or peptides). These are called *neurotransmitters*.

2. The dendrites of another neuron have specific *receptors* for each type of neurotransmitter. These receptors are usually proteins found in the structure of the cell wall which, when they come into contact with

neurotransmitters (for example, those emitted by the previous neuron through its axon terminal), produce a movement of ions and, consequently, a flow of electricity through the dendrites to the axon terminals of that neuron. One way to visualise what goes on in this phase is to imagine that if the electrical signal flows in the same direction as that of recent synapses, it is known as *excitation* (the total electricity flow increases). If, on the other hand, the electrical signal flows in the opposite direction, it is known as *inhibition* (the total electricity flow decreases).

3. When the electrical flow reaches the end of the axon, it triggers the release of new neurotransmitters through the axon terminals. These neurotransmitters cross the small divide between the axon terminal and the dendrites of another neuron, thereby initiating the cycle again and creating a new connection.

The process described above is a mere simplification of one isolated synapse in one single cell. In real terms, this activity activates thousands of diminutive molecules acting as neurotransmitters and, as a process, is replicated countless times. One single neuron is capable of forming between 1,000 and 10,000 synapses, weaving an intricate web with an enormous amount of cells. In short, if we remember that there are eighty billion or so neurons in our brain and factor them into the equation, we are left with a set of figures which is, quite simply, immense. In fact, we could say that the magnitude of what goes on in our brain is as enormous as it is difficult to really take in.

As each individual neuron has its own particular specialisation and, as such, is involved in very specific neuronal processes, each one forms excitatory and/or inhibitory synapses relatively infrequently. Speech, sight, hearing, recognising a face, identifying a smell, enjoying a particular taste, moving a muscle... indeed, this issue of neuron specialisation has given rise to a range of myths and misunderstandings about the brain, such as the popular belief that we only use one tenth of our brain's capacity. This is completely false. We use all of our brain, albeit part by part, in much the same way as we use all the muscles in our body but not all of them at the same time. That wouldn't really make much sense! We only need to look at those cases in which a small area of the brain has been damaged due to an accident or illness (cases which invariably result in some kind of negative consequence for one of the body's motor, cognitive or physiological functions) to see that this is so. If it were true that we really used such a small percentage of our brain, most cases of brain damage would have no lasting consequences.

However, the electrochemical flow described above does not only take place between one neuron and another but also between neurons and the different nerves and muscles spread throughout our body. This whole process is, therefore, not just a question of interneuronal communication but can also be considered as the fundamental *modus operandi* of the brain, of its communication system and its control over the human organism. It is this cerebral process that governs each and every one of our actions, conscious or otherwise, that regulates our body down to the finest detail and decodes external impulses received through our senses, giving rise to our corresponding responses.

In this respect, it should be emphasized that neurons work together as a team to perform all these functions, joining up in local groups and creating divisions and subdivisions in the brain. All those neurons involved in the same type of function are closely grouped together and coordinated to deliver a harmonious and coherent energy flow.

But it doesn't stop there. In addition to controlling, ordering and coordinating every single part of our body, neurons play another role that can only be described as extraordinary. The net result of all those myriad connections gives rise to the most spectacular, wondrous and inexplicable effect known to man: our perception of reality. That is... how we interpret our environment, visual decoding, listening and understanding, speech, reading, emotions, thoughts and consciousness. What you feel, reflect on and decide. In short, what you "are" is the result of this infinite, microscopic and truly sensational neural dance.

It's not easy for us to fully grasp and accept the implications of all these ideas. We are so caught up in our interpretation of reality that we don't realise that it really is nothing more than that: an interpretation, formed and governed by our brain. The fact that we consider everything around us as specific, definite and real is rooted in this, but scientific evidence is steadily revealing that reality is something much more complex and bizarre, something that goes far beyond our powers of comprehension. For example, in the realm of subatomic particles, very high energy environments or at the bottom of black holes, the way things happen is so unattached from our reality that it is practically impossible for us to imagine what goes on.

The following is an example that goes some way towards explaining the implications referred to above and what the brain is capable of. When you look around and see the range of colours that surround you, you need to understand that what you are experiencing is nothing more than an illusion. Why? Because colours, in themselves, do not exist. Colours are nothing more than a trick of the brain that enables us to discern the interval of electromagnetic radiation of the visible spectrum (in other words, of natural or artificial light) reflected or emitted by any given object. We call this "colour". It's likely that over time our ancestors developed this ability to see colour to distinguish between factors essential for their survival, e.g. the ripeness of certain fruits or the toxicity of certain vegetables.

Another engaging example of how our brain decodes information on objects around us is face identification, for which there is a specific and specialised area within the brain. To date, no artificial system has proved itself capable of equalling the capacity, speed and versatility of the human brain to distinguish and interpret a specific face among a multitude of faces. The most curious aspect of this is that it doesn't perform this feat by considering the face as the sum of a series of component elements (eyes, mouth, nose, etc.) but as a whole, converting the process into something emotional. That's why we say that we think a certain face looks familiar or not, and recognise a face immediately if we've seen it before, because we associate it unconsciously with a personality, with a possible conduct or behaviour.

The main reason why evolution has afforded us this ability is probably to anticipate the extent to which we can trust that person. Sometimes we get it right, other times we form ill-conceived prejudices but, in any case, the sight of a face suggests many things, mostly related to our feelings: in short, the brain makes us a finely-tuned machine for reading, identifying and classifying faces. Conversely, the effects of cerebral malfunction in this area of the brain are striking. People with brain damage in this area suffer from prosopagnosia, a condition which impairs face recognition as sufferers only perceive a face as the sum total of its component parts (eyes, nose, mouth, etc.). In other words, they do not recognise the face and are incapable of distinguishing someone, even a close relative, just by looking at their face. They can't even recognise their own face!

In any case, these are just two examples to illustrate the creative and interpreting capacity of the brain. Don't get me wrong: in providing you with these examples, I'm not suggesting that reality doesn't exist or that the universe and all that surrounds us is merely an illusion. The last thing I want is for you to confuse these ideas with those fanciful theories about parallel dimensions and imaginary worlds based on beliefs and myths, those ideas that use pseudoscientific arguments to supposedly justify what they propose. There can be no doubt that reality is there in front of us, that the mountains we know exist, that we relate to and with the people around us and that we're surrounded by sounds. What's important to understand is that the perception we have of all this is generated in our brain, that it's the brain that masterfully puts all these things together and creates that amazing story that each one of us considers to be our own reality. If we could replicate the neural activity generated by taking a walk through the woods, we wouldn't be able to distinguish that replica from the original sensation caused when that activity was really performed. In fact, we do this every night when we sleep. Dreams are nothing more than energy flows generated by our neurons, probably due to biochemically required processes of memory storage, cleansing and recharging. And while that energy is flowing, it brings to life an infinite number of abundantly detailed experiences.

The thing is, those experiences really only exist inside of us.

A neural jigsaw puzzle

From a functional and structural perspective, it's fair to say that the brain is really a type of jigsaw puzzle, the basic units of which are neurons but which, as I have mentioned before, is also made up of components of a higher order. These other components are groups of cells specialised in specific tasks and known as *brain areas*.

One example of this is the *brain stem*, located in the lowest part of the brain at the junction with the spinal cord. This area controls certain functions which are essential and basic for our existence, such as breathing, our heartbeat and digestion. In the inner brain, just above the brain stem, is the *hypothalamus*, one of the areas of most interest to us throughout this book as it manages aspects such as thirst, body temperature, sexual desire, hunger and satiety. Functions linked to instinct are found on the next level; for example, emotions such as fear and anxiety are managed in the amygdala, and the nearby hippocampus contains all the information required to store long-term memory.

Though most animal brains have many of the same or similar functional areas, the differences between species are appreciable and even greater and more relevant when comparing different classes of animal such as insects, reptiles or mammals. Originally, the brains of the most basic living creatures were composed exclusively of the most "automatic" brain areas (those which control the essential automatic body regulation mechanisms mentioned above). However, over the course of time, a series of layers of groups of neurons performing more complex and advanced functions have been added on top of those more basic areas. These neurons have accumulated in successive layers to form the cerebral cortex. The whole of this outer layer also houses functional areas, in this case called *lobes*, which also contain neurons involved in specialised activities usually related to conscious and more sophisticated and subtle processes such as audio and visual interpretation, speech, writing, conscious movements, abstract thought, consciousness and emotions, amongst others.

Another well-known myth is that our brain is divided into two halves (known as hemispheres and joined by the corpus callosum), one of which controls our rational side whilst the other controls our more emotional side. Anatomically speaking, it's true that our brain is divided into two very symmetrical parts, so this myth is rooted in a certain logic. Furthermore, in the past – based on evidence from accidents and neurosurgery – certain brain functions that could justly be classified as rational or emotional were attributed to one side of the brain or the other. However, technological developments that now enable us to visualise brain activity more precisely have revealed that the two hemispheres and the functional areas are interconnected on a massive scale, and that classifying certain functions as emotional or rational and attributing them to one or another of the cerebral hemispheres was not based on strong scientific evidence and could even be considered as incorrect.

As the brain is probably the most complex and sophisticated structure in the known universe (many experts consider it as such on the basis of our current knowledge of the universe), understanding its anatomy and the details of how it works is an incredibly difficult task which will keep neuroscientists occupied for some time to come. Everything you've read in these last few pages can therefore be considered as mere tenuous brushstrokes on the canvas of this eventual body of knowledge, intended to help you understand all the ideas we'll be looking at in future chapters of this book. In any case, for now, we have no need to go into the subject any further.

Neurology will no doubt come up with many more surprises and provide us with answers to many issues relating the brain with our body and our mind. In fact, we won't have to wait too long for these answers because it's already providing them, especially so in recent years, bringing to light an assortment of hugely intriguing concepts and ideas which will open up new and exciting medical perspectives.

And new and exciting perspectives on food and obesity.

REFERENCES

We Are Our Brains: A Neurobiography of the Brain, from the Womb to Alzheimer's (Swaab, 2011)

Amygdala Responsivity to High-Level Social Information from Unseen Faces (Freeman et al, 2014)

Response of face-selective brain regions to trustworthiness and gender of faces (Mattavelli et al, 2012)

An Evaluation of the Left-Brain vs. Right-Brain Hypothesis with Resting State Functional Connectivity Magnetic Resonance Imaging (Nielsen et al, 2014)

1.2. THE ENERGY REGULATOR

.

Let's get back to neurology. As mentioned in the previous chapter, the hypothalamus, though only approximately the size of a cherry, plays a key role in the brain. Widely researched and mapped, the hypothalamus is located in the core of the brain and is subdivided into a number of nuclei with names which are not easy to remember: anterior, posterior, lateral, paraventricular, lateral preoptic, supraoptic, suprachiasmatic, ventromedial, arcuate, etc. Each one of these nuclei has been associated with functions as diverse as they are important.

However, a brief diversion. Before going any further into the hypothalamus itself, let's take a quick look at the concept of a thermostat, since this is an analogy I shall be making repeatedly in this book. All of us more or less know what a thermostat is... a device fitted with some kind of signal receiver (a temperature sensor) which, when a certain pre-set value is reached, opens or closes an electrical circuit. All fridges are fitted with a thermostat to trigger the cooling circuit when the temperature goes up, thereby ensuring the inside of the fridge is kept at the required cold temperature. An increasing number of taps and radiators are also being fitted with a thermostat for the comfort and stability they provide in ensuring a constant water and room temperature respectively, in line with the settings the user has previously established. This analogy will be widely used throughout this book. In fact, one of the most essential functions of the hypothalamus is very similar to that of a thermostat, since it is responsible for maintaining our organism at a constant temperature regardless of the external temperature. Furthermore, the hypothalamus is also responsible for determining our circadian rhythms, i.e. the body's sleeping and waking hours that enable us to rest and be active.

In all of this, the function of the hypothalamus that most interests us here is the one we could refer to as the "energy regulator". This is the function that controls our food intake to ensure energy is available at all times, maintaining a balance or *homeostasis*, as experts call it. Just as a thermostat regulates temperature, the hypothalamus does the same but with energy requirements. From an anatomical perspective, the nuclei which most clearly have been associated with energy regulation and food intake are the laterals, the ventromedial and the arcuate.

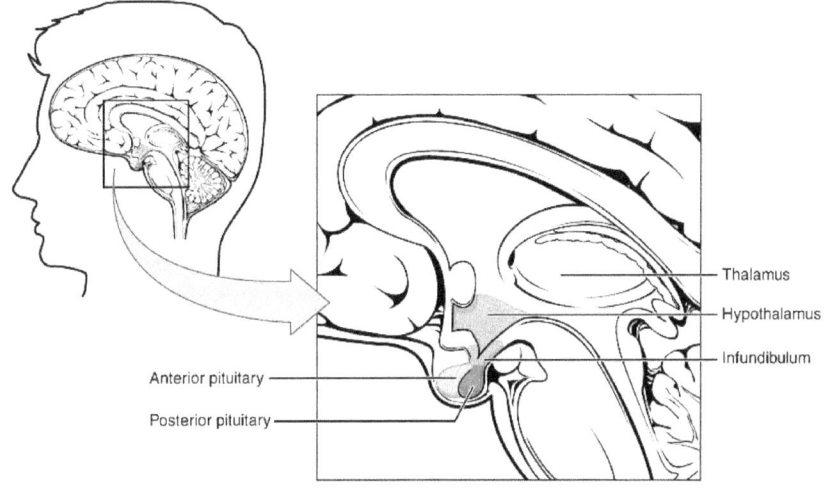

Location of the hypothalamus (Wikipedia- Anatomy & Physiology)

In short, this small mass of tissue is responsible, amongst several other things, for regulating exactly *when* and *how much* we have to eat, adjusting our desire to eat to the caloric requirements of our metabolism. In other words, it deals with energy in the same way as a thermostat deals with temperature, thereby triggering what we interpret as appetite (or hunger) and satiety (or fullness).

However, although this analogy of a thermostat may help us to understand the basics of how the hypothalamus works, exactly how it ensures that we eat all we need is rather more complex. It's relatively easy to perceive different ways of measuring room temperature or the temperature of an object but rather more difficult, even if you have been trained as a scientist, to imagine how consumption and the energy reserves of a living being can be measured.

The first studies relating this area of the brain to appetite were conducted over fifty years ago and carry a certain measure of prestige.

As is frequently the case in this type of studies, damaging the hypothalamus of laboratory animals enabled researchers to verify that hyperphagia (overeating) or hypophagia (undereating) can be provoked, depending on the specific area damaged. On the basis of these two independent effects, experts put forward the idea of a dual-point regulation system equipped, on one hand, with a centre for controlling satiety and, on the other, with a centre for controlling hunger. This hypothesis has mostly held true to date and has been confirmed by subsequent and more sophisticated experiments, as well as by studies on the consequences of damage to the human brain caused by disease or accidents.

At this point, it is important to understand that we are not talking about a system that increases or reduces caloric intake on the basis of one or two precise, simple and clear signals (as is the case with temperature). Metrics related to the energy expenditure of living beings are a much less obvious proposition. Furthermore, it should not be forgotten that this mechanism of caloric regulation is the product of millions of years of evolution. Through it, our metabolism is assured of something essential: that energy is available, and the presence, therefore, of a highly flexible and complex mechanism equipped with a wide range of multiple resources is to be expected. And this, effectively, is the case.

Initially, when scientists began looking into this field, the first theories or models of energy homeostasis (or balance) were rather simple. For example, the glucostatic model suggested that the energy balance was regulated by glucose levels in the blood. If the level of glucose was low, the hypothalamus would detect this and encourage us to eat: if levels were high, it would tell us to stop eating. However, we now know that although glucose levels are a quite reliable indicator to predict the beginning and end of meals, they struggle to provide us with answers if we attempt to correlate them with other relevant factors which impact significantly on the whole system such as accumulated fat and energy expenditure.

Years later, another model (commonly referred to as the lipostatic model) was put forward assigning body fat the role of generating the signals which activate or deactivate appetite to adjust energy input and expenditure. Studies in animals have confirmed that this model, though still overly elementary, is more accurate than the glucostatic model.

From mouth to hypothalamus

The fact that the hypothalamus is responsible (at least partially) for feeling the desire to eat or not, for triggering our resolve to dispel from our mind other thoughts and issues and to prioritise the urge to look for food, has been proven beyond doubt in many studies. However, the question is, what drives this reaction? What's the criterion for launching these orders? The temptation is to think that any decision we take to eat something put in front of us, to pick up a utensil and consume that food until we feel full, is a straightforward and obvious process, as it's something we do continuously and without any major complications, but this is not so. The neurobiology underlying this is extremely intricate and there are numerous processes and signals involved.

The passage of food through our body begins with the signals generated by our senses (sight and smell) which detect the presence of food. The characteristics of this food product are sent to the brain, where they are interpreted and processed for a decision to be taken. Our exceptional predictive capacity means it is not even necessary for us to see or smell the food directly: our prior and experiential learning enables a similar signal to be generated merely by perceiving something that reminds us of that food or of something we associate it with. This was demonstrated through the experiments of the Russian physiologist Ivan Pavlov with dogs, who began to salivate automatically whenever they heard the sound of the bell that Pavlov used to ring prior to feeding them. The brain then processes this information to decide whether it is time to eat or not, whether to order our muscles to pick up a spoon or whether to leave it for another time.

Once the food is actually in our mouth, its smell and texture are captured by sensors found in different parts of the inside of our mouth and nose. These sensors send signals to the frontal lobe of the brain, just above our eyes. This area of the brain, which is in constant interaction with the hypothalamus as we shall see in future chapters of this book, deciphers a wide array of smells and the different tastes we are capable of identifying. Furthermore, in conjunction with other areas of the brain, it is also responsible for producing that pleasurable feeling we get when we eat something we like, telling us the food in question is edible and most likely nutritious, whilst simultaneously controlling the activities of chewing, salivating and swallowing based on the information it receives on the physical properties (size, texture, etc.) of the food.

Immediately afterwards, during the process of digestion, a series of hormonal signals and flows are channelled through to the brain through the body's circulatory and nervous systems. These signals enable the brain to remain in control of the situation. The stomach is commonly believed to be a relatively simple and passive organ, where more or less previously-chewed food is received and where, thanks to gastric acids and enzymes, the real process of breaking down what we've eaten begins. However, experts have shown that the stomach is actually a very active, complex and versatile organ, with an abundance of nerves and sensors which capture and transmit information. More precisely, an enormous quantity of nerve fibres transmit nervous stimuli to the gastric mucosa and are able to detect locally secreted hormones. Hormones are chemical messengers which different parts of our body exchange to communicate some kind of message or to interact with each other. There is nothing particularly strange or unknown about them: they are relatively simple molecules synthesized by specialised cells of a diverse nature. Some hormones are derived from, or are chains of, amino acids (the basic units of proteins) whilst others are created from lipids and fats.

The principle behind this process of communication is, in theory, simple. The cells of a gland somewhere in our organism "send messages" by secreting hormones, which are transported in our circulatory system to make their way somewhere else. When they arrive to an area where there are cells with receptors which are sensitive to them, those receptors will detect them, the message will, so to speak, be "received" and, depending on the type of cell in question, a response or specific reaction will be triggered.

For example, leptin is a hormone produced in the fatty tissue which is closely related to the desire to eat: when leptin levels are high after we have eaten, it contributes to the feeling we have of being full. Conversely, ghrelin, discovered more recently and secreted by glands in the active gastric mucosa, has the opposite effect of stimulating the appetite.

After passing through the stomach, the food moves on to the intestine where, having now been reduced to its most basic components, it is progressively absorbed through the intestinal walls into the bloodstream. The mechanical movements of tension and release generate information which is sent to the brain but, as before, nerve fibres are also very active at this stage of digestion, transmitting chemical signals which once again are normally generated in the form of hormones. To give you an idea of what goes on, researchers have observed that at this stage of digestion, cholecystokinin (CCK) is secreted in the small intestine and peptide YY (PYY) and type 1 glucagon-like peptide (GLP-1) in the large intestine, all of which are considered to be appetite suppressants.

Finally, the nutrients which the digestive process has progressively been "selecting" pass through the intestinal wall into the circulatory system, where they are transported and distributed throughout the body and all our organs by the bloodstream. It is worth noting that they first pass through the liver, a type of super filter and mega-factory of components, where a large number of processes essential to our metabolism take place (we won't go any further into these for the moment). And throughout this process, the different sensors continue doing their work, detecting the presence of different elements such as glucose and hormones which may have been secreted by organs (for example, the pancreas) closely linked to gastrointestinal behaviour. Adipose tissue (stored fat) is in itself a complex organ and plays a highly active role in this system by secreting hormones in an effort to maintain its presence and thereby ensure that the body, if so required, can call on the necessary reserves of fat. Foremost amongst these hormones is leptin, which has a "direct line" to the brain and the hypothalamus.

At this point, I think it best to pause briefly in this express trip around our digestive and metabolic system to take another look, on a microscopic level, at what goes on inside our cells in their role as factories. Effectively, it is the "respiratory" mechanism of these incredible *nanomachines* that enables living beings to extract energy from foods.

We have seen that, through the actions of acids and enzymes, the digestive processes outlined above progressively break down the foods we eat and extract their essential components. In the case of foods with a high carbohydrate content (high-carb foods), the main product obtained is glucose, which is transported to all parts of the body through the circulatory system. When glucose molecules reach a cell, they can be visualized as passing through the cell membrane and, with the help of several components and chemical processes, penetrating into the cell itself. The first multi-reaction oxidation process, known as glycolysis, now begins inside the cell, during which various compounds are generated. The end-product of the process is pyruvic acid, or pyruvate.

Pyruvate now figures centrally in the process by entering the cell's mitochondria, the "oven" in which this small miracle is unfolding, and oxidising once again to produce another molecule, acetyl coenzyme A (or acetyl-CoA), which, as we shall see, is also destined to play a key role in the process.

Fatty acids (for example, from dietary fat or from adipose tissue) are also transported throughout the body in the bloodstream and may also reach cells. Having made their way into a cell using specific transporters, they too are oxidised in the cell's mitochondria (in a reaction known as beta oxidation), once again producing, amongst other things, molecules of acetyl CoA. This heralds the final stage, another sequence of reactions known as the Krebs Cycle or Citric Acid Cycle. Both pyruvate and acetyl CoA act as fuel during the initial stages of this complex series which generates two end products: carbon dioxide (CO_2) and water.

A summary outline of these processes is shown below:

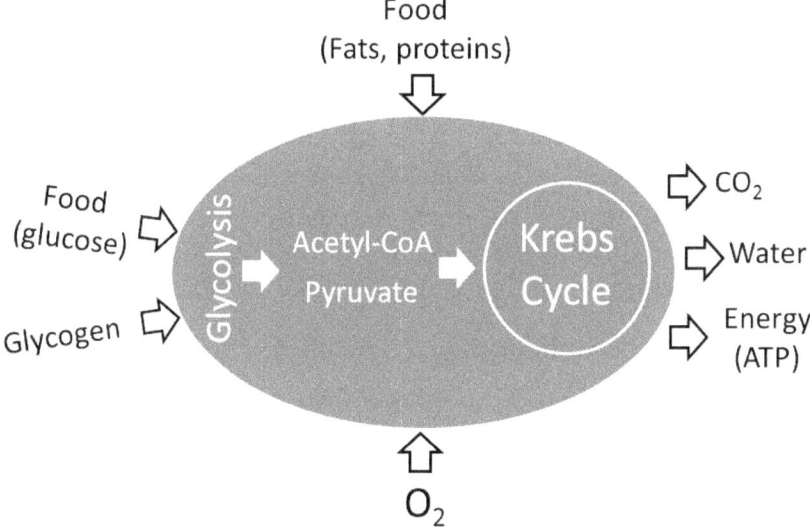

So where's the energy?

Several intermediate compounds are produced in the course of the different reactions and stages (glycolysis, Krebs cycle, etc.) mentioned above, one of which is adenosine triphosphate (better known as ATP). This is considered the basic unit of chemical energy. As ATP molecules are unstable in water (certain bonds of its atoms are weaker than the bonds formed with water), it converts relatively easily (through the process of hydrolysis) into another molecule, adenosine diphosphate (or ADP). When this occurs, a significant amount of energy is generated. It is this chemical energy which can be considered as the spark of life, as it is this energy that makes the cell "work" and which can be used as the driver of practically any other chemical reaction produced as part of the normal activity of our body.

Thus, we could say that a significant part of what happens inside us, in each and every one of the tiny units that make up our body, is chemistry driven by the vital impulses from hydrolysis of ATP molecules, and that those molecules have, in turn, been synthesized in the cell's mitochondria from different components of foodstuffs.

Amazing, don't you think?

What happens if the supply of glucose is neither perfect nor continuous? What will happen to the cells, particularly those who rely on this molecule for their functioning? What about if it's totally impossible to obtain food containing carbohydrates? So far, we have focused primarily on the metabolism of glucose but, as could be expected, our body is equipped with various alternative plans and mechanisms so as not to put all its eggs, so to speak, in one basket.

Let's look at them one by one:

1. Glycogen, the glucose storehouse. As we've seen, glucose is extracted from high-carb foods as part of the digestive process, absorbed into the bloodstream through the intestinal walls and subsequently transported around our body. Thus, plasma glucose (blood sugar) levels may vary significantly, depending on the time elapsed since the last time we ate and the use that has been made of that glucose. Fortunately, glucose can be stored in different parts of the body, especially in the liver and muscles, where it is structured in the form of branched linear chains known as glycogen. Glycogen is especially useful to ensure a constant and steady flow of glucose and the immediate availability of energy, since it acts as a buffer or regulator which our metabolism resorts to continuously.

2. Gluconeogenesis, the generation of glucose from proteins. As well as obtaining glucose directly from high-carb foods, our body can also call on another way to generate glucose to ensure its availability for certain cells which require it *sine qua non*. Both glucose and glycogen can be synthesised in various stages and reactions from the amino acids of proteins (taken, for example, from tissue or muscle) in a process known as gluconeogenesis. In the past, this mechanism was thought to be an exceptional, almost "emergency" resource of the body. However, it is now known to be operational at all times, and is especially active and of particular use in the absence of any external source of glucose, when the supply of reserve glycogen has been exhausted or if an extra supply of energy is required (for example, when following a low carbohydrate diet, fasting or in periods of strenuous exercise).

3. Acetil-CoA instead of glucose. If plasma glucose and glycogen reserves are finally exhausted and there is no external source of replenishment (though, as we have just seen, gluconeogenesis is always available to supply those cells with particular requirements for glucose), our metabolism changes its regular strategy for obtaining energy and switches to a type of "plan B", referred to by some experts as nutritional ketosis. In this case, molecules of acetyl-CoA, the same compound mentioned above as a post-glycolysis product, are generated from fatty acids (for example, from diet or accumulated fat). This compound can be used to produce so-called ketone bodies (more specifically, beta-hidroxybutyrate and acetoacetate) dispersed through the bloodstream. When these bodies come into contact with cells, they are once again converted, after a series of reactions, into acetyl-CoA. As we have seen before, this molecule acts as a nutrient in the Krebs Cycle and all its energy-generating reactions (ATP).

I appreciate that it's not easy to fully understand all these ideas if you are not familiar with these principles and this type of language. It's equally true that it is not essential for you to understand them perfectly to continue reading this book. However, I do think it's worth dedicating a few pages to explaining these ideas, as an understanding of the cellular energy metabolism of glucose, of lipids and of the three complementary energy mechanisms can provide us with a clear insight into how we obtain energy from foods.

In any case, more questions arise. For example, when and in what quantities do glucose molecules or fatty acids cross the cell membrane and oxidise? On what basis is the structural use of proteins and their participation in nucleogenesis prioritised? What criterion is used to decide whether fatty acids are stored or oxidised? How does the body maintain appropriate levels of glucose and fatty acids in the blood? On what basis is the decision taken to use muscle glycogen or plasma glucose? These and other such questions make it apparent that, in addition to a microscopic analysis of cells, a wider and more holistic perspective of the metabolism in general, as briefly described in earlier pages of this book, must be taken into consideration. Everything is modulated, regulated and controlled by an enormous quantity of subsystems and essential components (for example, the endocrine system, the digestive system, the brain, etc.), all of which together make up an intricate and, at least partially, still unknown network of interrelated and redundant systems.

At this point, I feel I should once again remind you that the descriptions above are a considerable simplification. Volumes of academic literature have been written on what science knows of the passage of food through our body and how energy is obtained from it. Nevertheless, returning to the main subject of this book and continuing in this line of simplification, I shall allow myself to further summarise the connection between all this metabolic activity and the control exerted by the brain, or more specifically the hypothalamus, in the following sentence:

"The neurons of the hypothalamus receive signals and information from our memory, our senses (images, smells, tastes), our organs, our digestive processes and our energy-generating metabolic processes, via the "messengers" (such as hormones) that run through our body".

Fine, but how is all this information interpreted? How do the neurons of the hypothalamus "read" this enormous quantity of signals generated in the process of eating, digesting and metabolising? As we saw a few pages ago, the dendrites of neurons have specific receptors which act as sensors capable of inter-reacting with specific stimuli, and the same is also true of the nerves that make up our nervous system. Our body contains thousands of millions of dendritic sensors continuously receiving signals, both in our brain cells and in the myriad and extensive branches of our nervous system that run to all corners of our body. Some molecules may come into direct contact with these brain cells after travelling around the body in the bloodstream and cross the barrier that isolates the brain and keeps it protected.

In any case, the receptor embedded in the wall of the cell's dendrites reacts to the presence of the hormone it is sensitive to, producing a biochemical response and a movement of ions which, in turn, creates a difference in electrical potential, or signal. This difference in potential is transferred through to the axon terminal where new neurotransmitters are released. Thus, a neural energy flow is created, distributed and exchanged among the different neurons throughout the functional area in question (in this case, the hypothalamus).

Even though these explanations may seem rather technical, I can assure you that you are very familiar with the final effect of all this electrochemistry. You know it as that feeling of hunger you get mid-morning, or when your stomach feels full after a big meal. This dual possibility of hunger-satiety can be explained by the existence of two types of neurons in the hypothalamus, or more precisely, in its arcuate nucleus: so-called NPY/AgRP neurons, which make us feel hungry when activated, and POMC neurons, which produce in us the feeling of being full. Both types of neuron take their strange names from the precursor molecules of the main neurotransmitter that they synthesize, and from the fact that, as neurons, they are equipped with more receptors of Agouti-related protein and Pro-opiomelanocortin, respectively (though recent studies have shown that these neurons may also be activated by the effect of other elements and specific hormones such as neuropeptide Y).

In other words, we could say that NPY/AgRP neurons are like switches which, when they connect, make you feel hungry, and that conversely, when POMC neurons connect, they make us feel full. So, it all comes down to a war of switches, the winner of which will be responsible for making us feel hungry or sated.

As you can see, even this simplified version of the reality of energy homeostasis is considerably more complicated than what the glucostatic and lipostatic models proposed. The truth is that the hypothalamus, that modest lump of neural tissue, is under constant bombardment by a multitude of food-related biochemical elements which stimulate or inhibit each one of its NPY/AgRP and POMC neurons.

The end result of which is the feeling (or not) of hunger.

As mentioned above, evolution and the passage of time have stabilised and developed this remarkably complex system into something powerful and redundant: that is to say, a system consisting of multiple solutions and processes to resolve any given problem, in such a way that if one process fails, others will step in to ensure the energy supply and balance, the energy homeostasis, is maintained. Remember: no energy, no life.

In which case, why does obesity exist? What's going wrong in this perfectly redundant energy regulator which has been so effective during millions of years? Or is it that this whole way of thinking about it is mistaken? Not completely, it would seem. Many of the proposals and theories that I've just outlined above have been soundly confirmed through careful and intensive research on both animals and humans. However, it would seem that this homeostatic and hypothalamus-related approach doesn't, in itself, provide us with all the answers. Evidence would suggest that more concepts need to be factored in to give us a more complete picture of the situation.

A new approach in which, once again, the brain plays a key role.

REFERENCES:

Taste, olfactory and food texture reward processing in the brain and obesity (Rolls, 2011)

Taste, olfactory and food texture reward processing in the brain and the control of appetite (Rolls, 2012)

Neurotransmitter in key neurons of the hypothalamus that regulate feeding behavior and body weight (Meister, 2007)

Neuroscience: Dissecting appetite (Trivedi, 2014)

The brain, appetite and obesity (Berthoud et al, 2008)

Obesity and Appetite Control (Keisuke et al , 2012)

The hypothalamic arcuate nucleus and the control of peripheral substrates (Amado et al, 2014)

Hypothalamic control of adipose tissue (Stefanidis et al, 2014)

The interaction between nutrition and the brain and its consequences for body weight gain and metabolism (la Fleur et al, 2014)

Genes and the hypothalamic control of metabolism in humans (Volckmar et al, 2014)

Peptides and food intake (Sobrino Crespo et al, 2014)

Neuroendocrine regulation of appetitive ingestive behavior (Rhinehart et al, 2013)

Neuroendocrine control of food intake (Valassi, 2007)

Neuronal control of energy homeostasis (Gao et al, 2007)

When do we eat? Ingestive behavior, survival, and reproductive success (Schneider et al, 2013)

The role of gut hormones and the hypothalamus in appetite regulation. (Suzuki et al, 2010)

The NPY/AgRP neuron and energy homeostasis (Morton et al, 2001)

1.3. EATING GIVES US PLEASURE

Compared with the shops of yesteryear, modern-day supermarkets offer an enormous quantity and diversity of food products capable not only of meeting the nutritional needs of just about anyone but also the most unexpected and sophisticated whims and vagaries of the most discerning palates.

However, this excess of products stands in stark contrast with the small number of companies responsible for their production. As we shall see in later chapters of this book, the production of food worldwide is concentrated in the hands of a few huge and well-known corporations. One of the basic principles on which all these corporations operate is customer focus: in other words, to include the desires and preferences of potential customers in all their production operations, especially product development, to be able to offer consumers the products they most appreciate. And all, of course, with the objective of maximizing sales and profits, the very reason for their existence.

Acutely aware of the importance of this issue, these companies assign a huge amount of resources to their processes of new product creation (and to renewing or improving existing products), with international teams of hundreds or even thousands of people highly skilled and experienced in the field of research and development. Later, of course, all these efforts are further reinforced by marketing and publicity, the basic tools used nowadays to promote, market and sell products.

As you can imagine, the process of creating a product of "interest" (normally in terms of profitability) is not easy at all for these companies. Before they even begin, those given responsibility for coming up with such a product must not only take into account several prior factors but also, for obvious reasons, the overall strategy of their particular company. Such strategies are established to help technicians draw up the right proposals and have themselves have been drawn up on the basis of key information compiled and prioritised by specialist experts whose remit is to identify both current and future consumer trends. This key information often includes dietary recommendations issued by official bodies, preferences and trends in flavours, components with a good or bad image, environmental impact, etc.

All this information, together with other factors such as cost and accessibility of raw material and the later need to optimise the industrial manufacturing processes involved, is then worked on by developers in their laboratories (at the end of the day, no more than high-tech versions of your kitchen at home). Particular, or even obsessive, attention is paid to aspects of food safety (these large companies take extreme care in this respect... they are all too aware of what's at stake if they make a mistake) until they reach the stage of the final prototypes of the product they have in mind.

Obviously, leading food companies are keen to minimize the possibility of new product failure, as this would represent a considerable financial loss. To do so, prior to their launch onto the market, products are put through a series of filters and tests which involve contrasting the manufacturer's opinion with that of other experts, marketing specialists and, especially, the opinion of the potential buyers of the product: the customers. Throughout the long and laborious process of product creation, panels of intermediate and end consumers, of both a general and specialised nature, are asked to rate a series of important aspects including, amongst others, price and format. However, one aspect is given particular and specific importance: the organoleptic characteristics of the product. This is the term experts use to describe the properties that our senses assign to a foodstuff: appearance, colour, taste, smell, flavour (the mixture of smell and taste), aftertaste, etc. Consumers are asked to use predetermined scales to score each of these properties which, at the end of the process, are given ultimate and primary importance in terms of product rating.

The outcome of all this is what is referred to as the *hedonic perception*, or put in simpler terms, a rating expressing *how much* potential customers like the product. If all other variables are considered to be within acceptable parameters, the final hedonic value may decide whether the company commits itself to the product and launches it definitively on the market.

The importance of consumers' hedonic perception should not come as a surprise to us: after all, it is consumers who will buy the product or not, depending on how much they like it (on the assumption, I repeat, that all the other aforementioned issues relative to price and other influencing variables are within acceptable parameters).

In short, the industry manufactures what we like and we eat it. Because we're hungry... or perhaps not.

Pleasure and health

This strategy is not exclusive to the food sector: all leading and competitive companies produce things that people want to buy. Car manufacturers, for example, produce cars at a wide range of prices which accentuate the thrill of driving and provide owners with a potential status symbol. Similarly, mobile phone manufacturers offer phones with a wide range of user-friendly functions, and clothes manufacturers supply us with affordable clothing in a myriad different designs and with a wide range of details. In short, articles which consumers like. So why should the food industry be any different?

Firstly, cars, mobile phones and designer clothes are in no way absolutely essential items, and we don't normally associate them with our health. It's true that driving a car with a mechanical problem or which has a mediocre safety system could prove fatal, handling a faulty electronic device could seriously injure us and manufacturing cheap clothing can be harmful to the environment. Nevertheless, these are all relatively low possibility and isolated risks posing little direct threat to our health and which, furthermore, are controlled by strict standards established over the years. Vehicle safety systems have dramatically reduced the number of fatalities in car accidents, devices which run on electricity must comply with very strict standards minimizing the possibility of electric shock or fire, and there has been a steady and progressive demand in developed countries for all types of production companies to control and reduce waste and implement and comply with environmental management systems.

In contrast, we need to eat to survive. We have to eat food every day, a lot of which is manufactured using complex transformation processes. If something goes wrong in these processes, the potential risks are much more real, immediate and large-scale than in the case of other types of products. The food we eat every day has a considerable and direct impact on our health. It may contain toxic or dangerous constituents but, in this respect, a big effort has been made over recent decades and the industry is particularly scrupulous in this issue. Most unwanted constituents are identified, and there is an abundance of legislation obliging companies to control and maintain the presence of these constituents below quite stringent safety levels. We can, therefore, safely say that the food we eat is safer than ever.

But safety is not the only issue to bear in mind when discussing health and food. In other areas, food manufacturers have, to date, practically been given open licence, with no restrictions or guidelines on what they develop. And in saying this, I'm referring to the concept of what "healthy eating" should be.

Let me explain the difference. Safe food is not necessarily healthy food. The problem is that the first of these two concepts, safety, is primarily concerned with toxicology, i.e. with possible short-term negative effects, usually assessed by conducting experiments and trials on animals. This is quite an effective method for identifying those elements which cause significant damage in relatively short periods of time, but diet is something we follow throughout our life and which, for obvious reasons, has a very long-term effect. It's also true, as mentioned above, that the so-called western diet has been proven to be safe and that it minimizes food poisoning. However, the reality of the world around us and findings of recent epidemiological studies would both seem to bear out the idea that this diet contributes little in helping us reach old age in the best possible health: for example, in preventing the proliferation of diseases such as obesity and diabetes.

Or, put another way, it's not as healthy as it could be.

In today's world, the responsibility for choosing a healthy diet is, unfortunately, mainly in the hands of each individual. Beliefs such as *"there are no good or bad foods"* and *"the important thing is one's dietary pattern, not individual foodstuffs"* are mantralike and deep seated in society, so the only obligation food manufacturers have in this respect is to pander to possible preferences and trends shown by consumers when choosing the products they buy, depending on the degree to which they have been educated in food. However, as we shall see in later sections of this book, educating people in this area has little chance of succeeding in the face of the heavy artillery of food marketing.

This last paragraph may have reminded you of those food labels with nutritional information and the traffic light system used to inform us of the nutritional content of foodstuffs. Doesn't this system provide us with information on how healthy a food is? Our first reaction may be to think it does, that this information may be of use for consumers to assess the health value of a food, especially by identifying the amount of nutrients in that food that, supposedly, it is recommended to reduce or control. But the reality is entirely different. Results of recent research challenge the validity of certain historical recommendations to reduce the intake of certain substances such as fats and proteins, whilst other findings indicate that, in real terms, all this information is practically useless for most people. In short, that basing the health value of any given foodstuff on nutritionism is of very little use.

All these ideas take on even more importance when we consider the amount of highly processed foods we eat. These foods have been completely transformed in terms of their original raw materials and we are, as yet, ignorant of the long-term effect of this on our health. A very high proportion of the regular diet of those of us living in the western world is based on this type of product. In fact, their presence in the western diet exceeds that of fresh products, accounting for up to 60% of total calorie intake. These products are readily available and theoretically safe in the short-term but many of them have been manufactured with one primary objective: to maximise our sensorial response and to provide the consumer with a very gratifying experience.

Thus, if the long-term health of the population is to be considered a key priority, answers to a series of fundamental questions must be found. For example, can the pleasure produced by eating technologically processed foods, a pleasure which is probably greater than that normally experienced when eating fresh or natural foods, have an impact on our eating habits and health? Could this have something to do with the epidemic of chronic diseases associated with obesity? Could this even be a crucial factor behind why we eat? And is it reasonable to leave the food sector to its own devices in terms of self-regulation in this area, responding exclusively to customer needs and expectations identified through their buying patterns?

To find the answers to these questions, I believe we must first delve a little deeper into how our brain "lives" this pleasure, or satisfaction, from a neurological perspective, and thereby get a better understanding of what some refer to as *hedonic eating*, complementing the theory of homeostatic eating that we have just looked at.

The reward system of the brain

In 2013, experts from the University of Alabama designed an assessment tool to illustrate the extent to which the reasons why we eat go beyond the acquisition of energy. The "Palatable Eating Motives Scale" consists of a questionnaire designed to identify the most common reasons and motives that induce us to eat those products we are especially fond of. The authors focused particularly on those foods commonly considered as most desirable and satisfying, i.e. sweets (chocolate, cookies, cake, candy, ice-cream, etc.), salty snacks (crisps, pretzels, crackers, etc.), fast food (hamburgers, cheeseburgers, pizza, fried chicken, chips, etc.) and sugary drinks (soft drinks, shakes, sweet tea or coffee, etc.).

The questionnaire included a list of the most-frequently identified reasons for consuming these foods and drinks. Respondents were asked to tick those options they believe correspond with their particular reasons. The options were:

1. To forget your worries

2. Because your friends want you to eat/drink them

3. Because it helps you enjoy a party

4. Because it helps you when you feel depressed or nervous

5. To be sociable

6. To cheer up when you are in a bad mood

7. Because you like the feeling

8. So that others won't kid you about not eating or drinking these items

9. Because it's exciting

10. To get "high-like" feelings

11. Because it makes social gatherings more fun

12. To fit in with a group you like

13. Because it gives you a pleasant feeling

14. Because it improves parties and celebrations

15. Because you feel more self-confident and sure of yourself

16. To celebrate a special occasion with friends

17. To forget about your problems

18. Because it's fun

19. To be liked

20. So you won't feel left out

As can be seen, not one of the reasons on this list is related to the energy balance or the need for nutrition. The results of the questionnaire enabled the experts to ratify that many of us very frequently decide to eat for emotional, social and psychological reasons... a perspective which is far removed from macronutrients and gross calorie counts. And what is responsible for this close relationship between eating and our emotions? The answer, undoubtedly, is our brain, that device responsible for managing both nutrition and feelings.

As we saw in the previous section speaking about energy homeostasis, the hypothalamus reacts to a myriad hormones and other such signals to ensure a sufficient supply of energy. However, if you're one of those people waging their daily personal war on excessive appetite and battling against the odds to keep yourself from being overweight, everything you read in that part may well have sounded very theoretical and far from your reality. When you think about your body (which perhaps is not as perfect as you'd like it to be and maybe has an excess of accumulated fat), it may be difficult for you to imagine it as a perfect piece of machinery, like that precise and redundant multiple *energy regulator* we spoke about before. All that information about sensors and receptors capturing signals and relaying them to the hypothalamus for them to be decoded to modulate your feeling of fullness. All this may be part of the original design, of what's evolved over millions of years, but for some people this is a mere idyllic utopia and, quite simply, just doesn't add up. If that energy thermostat worked as it should do, we wouldn't eat if we didn't need to and obesity wouldn't exist.

Furthermore, neither do we live or generally perceive this issue as being something unconscious and automatic. For example, we all perceive eating as being something much less simple than breathing, which is also, like eating, a process of introducing external elements into our body for them subsequently to be incorporated into our metabolism. We all know what it's like to feel breathless and what the quick and immediate answer to it is: take a deep breath. No healthy person decides to hyperventilate without good reason; we don't sit down with our family or friends to "have some breaths" together; none of us arrange to get together with some friends to breathe and talk about old times; nobody tries to drown their sorrows by taking a few breaths of fresh air.

Think about those just-baked croissant rolls you eat at the weekend for breakfast, or those chocolates you pick at now and again which are stashed away in a box at the bottom of the cupboard in the living-room. Think about your favourite pizza, that one you could easily eat on your own in one go even though it's family-sized. It's clear that many of us take special enjoyment from eating these foods, despite the fact that we may feel guilty afterwards if we've eaten too much. The key to the differences between what we feel when we eat and what we feel when we breathe is, once again, in our brain. Because eating, apart from nourishment and energy, gives us pleasure.

Though experts fully acknowledge the role played by the hypothalamus in controlling the energy flowing in and out of our body, i.e. that it responds to the myriad different signals it receives and thereby modulates our basic feelings of being hungry or feeling full, they have also been aware for some time that it is not the only part of our brain involved in controlling what we eat. Research conducted on both animals and persons has shown that many things happen between the moment we first smell the presence of a food and the period, after eating it, of digestion. During this time, our brain reacts and responds in many ways and in areas beyond the hypothalamus. Modern-day techniques of neurological screening have confirmed these ideas and provided us with information on the key role of a particular and essential concept in eating behaviour: *brain reward*.

In scientific terms, brain reward refers to the feeling of pleasure or positive motivation felt as the consequence of a particular action. In all probability, brain reward is a powerful tool which has evolved over time in human beings to encourage us to behave in a certain way which is beneficial for our survival and which, at the same time, is rooted in something very basic, simple and highly effective as an element of persuasion: the generation of a positive feeling as a reward for a specific behaviour. This is known by psychologists as *positive reinforcement*.

The perfect example of this is sexual pleasure, an unquestionably highly convincing and effective resource for practising intercourse and ensuring reproduction of the species. It is unnecessary here to explain how we feel sexual attraction, how we like to observe those individuals we find attractive and how our brain rewards us when we engage in sex. However, the reward system goes quite some way beyond an orgasm: it has many nuances and, in reality, is not just one single thing. In fact, from a scientific perspective, the concept has no precise definition. Indeed, even experts themselves sometimes intermix the terms reward, pleasure and motivation, and I personally believe there is still some way to go before a strong consensus on this issue is reached. In terms of each individual's subjective perception of them, these concepts may seem quite distinct from each other (we often talk of happiness, enjoyment or satisfaction), but they are not at all easy to pin down following more objective and neurological criteria.

In any case, it is not my intention here to go any further into this, as this insight into eating and pleasure does not require any greater degree of detail. In short, we can summarise by saying that our brain provides us with a variety of pleasurable sensations which are commonly considered as different versions or components of what is understood as reward. An orgasm, the feeling we experience when we feel loved by someone we love and witnessing a spectacular sunset are all good examples of the degree of sophistication of our neurons in this area. And, of course, a good meal is another example. Various areas of the brain are involved in these reward-related sensations, and those same areas are interlinked to form the so-called *reward circuit*. In the case of food, most of these areas are in the lower front part of our brain, near the hypothalamus.

What follows is a brief and summarised description of the functions of these areas. The orbitofrontal cortex and the amygdala encode information on food reward values. The insula processes information related to food taste and its hedonic evaluation. The nucleus accumbens and the dorsal striatum, receiving signals from the ventral tegmental area and the substantia nigra, regulate the motivational and incentive properties of foods. The lateral hypothalamus can regulate reward responses (what makes food appealing) and drives the motivation to go looking for food.

As you can see, the reward circuit is complex (as are the terms associated with it, a common feature of neurology), and consists of a system of intricate interconnections which functions in a way we do not, as yet, fully understand. Microscopic observation of these areas reveals they are composed of neurons, just like the other areas of the brain. In this case, the neurotransmitter mostly used by the neurons is dopamine, which will feature heavily in the rest of this chapter as it plays a key role in the brain's reward system and its consequences.

At this point, it is worth pointing out that any food we especially like and which brings about a pleasurable sensation in us is commonly referred to in academic terms as being a *high palatability* food. However, it must also be said that, to date, there is no great volume of scientific literature on which foods and isolated ingredients activate, to a greater or lesser degree, these areas of the brain; in other words, those foods which are more or less palatable. A series of individual experiments have been conducted, though these were focused more on neurobiological research than on nutritional components, so what we know on this matter is, at this moment in time, of a rather generic nature. There is a fair amount of consensus on the idea that sugar and fat are the components which most contribute to this characteristic in foods, though as any experienced cook or researcher in the food sector knows only too well, other strategically used ingredients and textures may also achieve outstanding results in this respect.

Recent research comparing the effect of fats to that of sugar reveals a marked response of the reward circuit to sweet foods. Furthermore, this response becomes greater as the quantity of this component increases: the more sugar, the greater the pleasure. However, in the case of fats, pleasure would seem to peak once a certain quantity or percentage has been reached in the fat composition of the food in question: however much fat may be added after that point, no greater pleasure is experienced.

Other variables also impact on palatability. For example, each individual's eating history plays a major role, as the foods we have eaten most often in the past impact on our preferences and on perceived palatability.

Reward, decision making and dopamine.

We have seen that pleasurable foods trigger a special effect in our reward circuit, and that neurons are at the core of the operational system of that circuit. In other words, that we eat not only to obtain energy but also because we like to. However, one essentially critical moment in the whole process remains unaddressed: the decision making moment, or the neurological process involved when we feel the urge to get up from wherever we are to go to the fridge, take a specific food and eat it. This action, if repeated frequently, becomes a habit, and research into human habits, including eating habits, ushers in one of the most complicated questions to find an answer to: the reasons underlying this habit. This is an essential issue to look into if we are to get to the root of the problem, so let's take a look at it now.

As explained in a previous chapter of this book, neurotransmitters are the chemicals through which information is transmitted from one neuron to another. That is, neurotransmission activates receptors which trigger a potential difference in the cell and, consequently, a power flow is generated. From previous chapters of this book, you will know by now that this, in a simplified and summary form, is the basis of brain activity.

Dopaminergic neurons are those which excite and generate this power flow, principally using dopamine as a neurotransmitter. What's more, as you may by now have surmised, the cells making up the reward circuit are mostly of this type, activated principally by dopamine. The importance of dopamine in the brain's reward system was discovered by James Olds and Peter Milner in the 1950s. These two brain researchers observed that rats came back time and again to an area of their cage where they were given a small electric current using an electrode implanted into their brain. This reaction led the researchers to deduce that this small electric discharge produced pleasure in the animals. As other scientists were later to confirm, what this current was actually provoking was the secretion of dopamine.

Prof. Wolfram Schultz, a neuroscientist at the University of Cambridge, has since become a reference on the relationship between dopamine and reward. His initial experiments with monkeys, conducted in the 1970s and 80s, enabled him to discover key aspects of this neurotransmitter. A little more in-depth knowledge of these experiments may help us to understand the interesting implications of the findings of his research.

One of his best-known experiments was conducted as follows. Firstly, Schultz produced a clearly audible sound, and a few seconds later, he poured apple juice into the monkeys' mouths. Throughout this experiment, the brain activity of the animals was being monitored using electrodes implanted in their brains. The neuroscientist observed that initially, dopaminergic neurons were only activated after the monkeys had received the juice, thereby triggering the feeling of reward. However, once this same operation had been repeated several times, the same neurons began to be activated in the monkeys just by hearing the sound produced beforehand, prior to the animals actually receiving the juice. In other words, neuronal activity was being triggered by expectation of reward, without actually waiting for the reward to come about as a consequence of the corresponding sensory signals of taste and smell. Or, put another way, the neurons were displaying predictive behaviour: not only were they being activated by the act of eating but also by anticipating it.

So, what do all these experiments have to do with the decision-making process that leads us to eat something we consider to be desirable? In short, a lot. This phenomenon of predictive behaviour has a sensory impact on the monkeys' reality... and, of course, on that of us humans, as well. The premature release of dopamine and the activity of the corresponding neurons triggers an emotional state which may well be very familiar to you: the expectation of reward and a motivation, a strong motivation, to go and find it... at whatever cost. And you feel this way because that premature release of dopamine, and the consequent neuronal activity it triggers, translates, in the biochemical parlance of the brain, as "*I want to do whatever's necessary to get that reward*". And you, within the parameters of your reality and immediate environment, interpret (and feel) that message that way.

When you actually get to eat that food that has excited your neurons so much, dopamine will once again be released and you will feel a sense of satisfaction. On the other hand, if you don't actually get around to eating that food and your dopaminergic circuit is left wanting, predictive dopamine will continue to be secreted and your brain will interpret this in a way you probably know only too well: that uncomfortable and unpleasant feeling of frustration.

So, as you can see, dopamine plays a key role in this decision-making process and, on a more general level, in the correct operation of our neurons. Indeed, its considerable and extensive importance in relation to brain activity, coupled to its relation with various neurological diseases such as Alzheimer, have led to an abundance of research on dopamine in recent decades. Though new studies have shown that other neurotransmitters, such as opioids and serotonin, are also involved in the reward circuit, these findings need to be further defined through more research work. Conversely, the relevance of the activity of dopamine in many areas of the brain associated with emotion, and particularly with the reward circuit, is very clear and better-known.

Why we eat

Everything you have read in the chapter above refers to decision-making from a biochemical and neuronal perspective. Such a decision-making process could be associated with instinctive reactions generated by quite basic primary signals. However, are all our decision-making processes of this same type? What about those decisions taken after careful consideration?

As humans, we tend to believe that we are rational beings capable of making a reasonably objective assessment of the pros and cons of a given situation prior to taking a particular decision. However, from a neurological perspective, things are not so clear-cut. Findings from recent research and experiments would indicate that, rather than logical analysis and reasoning, it is very often the emotional perspective that ultimately sways us towards one option or another. In fact, the process of reflection can often be considered almost as a mere justification for a decision that has already been taken intuitively and unconsciously. This has been confirmed by studies on brain damage. People who have suffered some kind of brain damage affecting their dopaminergic activity have difficulty in feeling emotions such as fear, anxiety and anguish, as well as in taking decisions. There are many documented cases of patients of this type whose analytical and logic skills are intact but who are incapable of living a minimally normal life because it is practically impossible for them to take a simple decision that, for anyone else, would be taken almost automatically.

Some researchers have reached surprising conclusions in the field of decision-making through conducting a series of simple and clear experiments. One such experiment involves asking the research subject to take a simple decision; for example, *"what shall I drink, an orange juice or an apple juice?"*, or any such everyday choice very similar to those we make when we decide whether to eat or not or to eat one thing in preference to another. Just by observing the activity of the brain in these cases, scientists are able to predict the decisions which are going to be taken before the research subjects consciously take them. And yes, you've read that right. The decision that is going to be taken can be predicted just by monitoring brain activity, and even before the decision-maker him/herself has actually taken it!

In addition to posing important questions in relation to an individual's free will, the findings of this revolutionary research also confirm once again that the decision whether to eat or not is not so much rational as something highly automatic, instinctive and emotional. In which case, does willpower exist? And whatever happened to reasoning, that factor which, above all others, distinguishes us from other animals? How does all this square up with our logically thought-out ideas regarding whether we should eat a given foodstuff or not?

Well, don't worry... the capacity of your brain to reason hasn't disappeared! Long-term planning and reflective analysis are conducted from the prefrontal cortex of the brain, a fine layer of neurons located at the front of the head just above your eyes, on a level with your forehead. Compared with that of our prehistoric ancestors, this is the part of our head which has evolved the most, with modern craniums revealing a pronounced bulge which can be seen to be progressively more sunken the farther back in time we go. Neurologically, this part of the brain is connected to many other areas and enables us to come up with answers to questions, as it has the capacity to analyse and resolve complex issues. These myriad connections enable the content of those areas to be consulted, such as the areas related to memory which house an enormous quantity of stored information. Depending on our previous knowledge and experience of any given issue, i.e. on the volume and precision of the "data file" we have on that issue, this network of connections relays this information, to a greater or lesser degree, for us to conduct the in-depth analysis required.

And how exactly are the activities of the prefrontal cortex coordinated with, or linked to, dopaminergic neurons, the reward system and everything else we've just been looking at? Let me give you a simple example, directly related to the subject of this book, to try to explain.

Imagine you go to a buffet restaurant for dinner. When you arrive, you see you've been presented with two options for the first course: one, a delicious dish of pasta in a tempting meat and tomato sauce with grated cheese on the top, and the other, a fresh and colourful mixed salad served with a copious amount of dressing. You look at both dishes several times and give your decision a moment's thought. Or, at least, that's what you think you do.

Certain studies have concluded that the decision you're going to take can be predicted just by analysing the amount of time you spend looking at one dish or the other. This is quite reliable as a pointer to the decision you're about to take, as we normally and unconsciously spend longer looking at those foods we associate with more rewarding hedonic feelings.

In any case, your brain clicks into gear and starts the decision-making process. On one hand, depending on how long it's been since you last ate and on your need for energy, your hypothalamic neurons will begin to emit signals to choose the option which contains more or less calories. On the other hand, the reward-related areas of your brain will also be activated on a significant scale, pre-empting the possible different senses of pleasure that either or both of the dishes may provoke in you, especially the pasta dish with the wonderful tastes its ingredients have to offer. If you don't like one of those ingredients, then the insula, a part of the brain responsible for sending inhibitory signals, may also come into play.

At the same time as all this, the prefrontal cortex will also be activated, gathering information from, and networking with, other areas of the brain, particularly those related to memory, to analyse and assess the pros and contras of each option and squaring all this data up with what you personally know about nutrition, your own personal objectives, your ideals and your principles.

Energy, desire and reason. Need, pleasure and logic. Three different perspectives, three different viewpoints colliding and overlapping each other amidst the neuronal interconnections of the brain. If your body has an urgent need for energy, the orexin neurons (those which provoke appetite) in the hypothalamus will be in full swing and will drive you towards choosing the dish with the highest calorific value. If your reward circuit is particularly attracted by the feelings that a big dish of pasta triggers in you, it will be awash with dopamine to win the battle. Conversely, if you have firm ideas about nutrition or your doctor has forbidden you to eat this type of food because of a serious health problem you may have, you'll bite the bullet and your prefrontal cortex will battle on bravely. In the end, you'll definitively choose one option or the other, either pasta or salad, depending on who wins this biochemical battle.

If we could see what goes on in the brain in these moments, what we'd probably see is that the area of the brain which is most intensely activated wins the battle. In doing so, and once again by networking with other areas, the winning area sends out the corresponding "orders" to trigger the cascade of signals that mobilises the rest of your organism, culminating in you stretching out your arm to pick up the chosen first course.

The way our brain resolves this neuronal horse-trading, whatever the end result may be, is quite remarkable. If reasoning wins the day, you will be capable of ignoring the messages the hypothalamus and areas of the reward circuit will likely still be sending, and you will opt for the salad. However, if your "instinct" eventually wins the day, pleasure will prevail over prudence and the pasta dish will be the chosen one, thereby calling into question the prefrontal cortex, the precursor to human reasoning. But never fear... your brain also knows how to deal with this discrepancy. Research has revealed that in these cases, the prefrontal cortex remains highly active but busies itself with a different issue altogether: it looks for reasons to justify the decision taken by its "rival", our instinct. In other words, what could be described as an ex post facto analysis. Returning to our original example, if you choose the pasta dish, your prefrontal cortex will probably come up with arguments to explain this decision (*"it's only for today, I need the energy because I'm not feeling 100%, I've had a bad day and I need something to cheer me up, etc."*). For you, those arguments will seem very persuasive.

This phenomenon of self-justification is very well known and has been widely studied in psychology. You too will have seen it in action quite often when listening to people trying to reason through their peculiar arguments on particularly sensitive issues such as politics, religion and relationships. The main aim of this mechanism is to reduce what is known as cognitive dissonance. Our brain needs to reduce its internal stress and controversies to continue functioning normally, and we all clearly, though unconsciously, tend to use reasoning and logic for one specific purpose: to preserve existing ideas and previously-taken decisions instead of remaining open to new perspectives on them.

The brain and obesity

So, in this first part of the book, I have outlined how the brain and its basic units (neurons) work and gone into a little more detail regarding how the brain controls and manages our food intake. This second question has been analysed from two different perspectives: on one hand, energy homeostasis, and on the other, hedonic feelings, i.e. those related to satisfaction and pleasure.

Having established this theoretical framework, I believe we are now in a position to begin talking about obesity. Though we have at no point veered off the subject of food, we have yet to address the main issue of this book (and probably the one that first made you take the decision to read it): the epidemic of overweight and obesity.

In the chapters that follow, this issue will be tackled head-on. However, throughout what follows, the key player will once again be a figure which doesn't normally crop up in this type of battle.

The brain.

REFERENCES

Profiling motives behind hedonic eating. Preliminary validation of the Palatable Eating Motives Scale (Burgess et al, 2013)

Consumption of ultra-processed foods and likely impact on human health. Evidence from Canada (Moubarac et al, 2014)

Hedonic and incentive signals for body weight control (Egecioglu et al, 2011)

Relative ability of fat and sugar tastes to activate reward, gustatory, and somatosensory regions (Stice et al, 2013)

Ghrelin and Dopamine: New Insights on the Peripheral Regulation of Appetite (Abizaid, 2009)

The Roles of Dopamine and Serotonin in Decision Making: Evidence from Pharmacological Experiments in Humans (Rogers, 2011)

Time of conscious intention to act in relation to onset of cerebral activity (readiness-potential). The unconscious initiation of a freely voluntary act (Libet et al, 1983)

Unconscious determinants of free decisions in the human brain (Haynes et al, 2008)

How we decide (Lehrer, 2010)

Reward mechanisms in obesity: new insights and future directions (Kenny, 2011)

Relation of obesity to consummatory and anticipatory food reward (Styce et al, 2009)

Energy regulatory signals and food reward (Figlewizc et al, 2010)

Appetite control and energy balance regulation in the modern world: reward-driven brain overrides repletion signals (Zheng et al, 2011)

Liking vs. wanting food; importance for human appetite control and weight regulation (Finlayson, 2007)

Decision making and the brain: Neurologist view (Pirtosek, 2009)

Elaborated Intrusion Theory: A Cognitive-Emotional Theory of Food Craving (May et al, 2012)

Methylphenidate decreases fat and carbohydrate intake in obese teenagers (Danilovich et al, 2014)

Dopamine Modulates the Neural Representation of Subjective Value of Food in Hungry Subjects (2014)

The presence of real food usurps hypothetical health value judgment in overweight people (2016)

PART 2

A MALADJUSTED BRAIN

As mentioned in the Introduction to this book, I'm taking it for granted you are aware that obesity is a worldwide problem. The upward trend in obesity is generally reflected in the mass media, whilst endless campaigns to combat it are launched and fade away, one after the other, in countries around the world, generally to little avail due to popular indifference.

Though economic development offers many advantages, we are slowly discovering that it also has some negative effects. One of these is the problem of becoming overweight, a kind of side effect of wealth occurring worldwide and which, to date, we have not been able to neutralise. Just the opposite, in fact: its rise is inexorable, reaching levels of real concern. As a result, related healthcare expenditure has shot up, quality of life is, for many, on a downward curve (especially among the elderly) and evidence points to the possibility that it may even be jeopardising the sustained increase in life expectancy enjoyed by mankind in recent decades.

In historical terms, the fact is that this high prevalence of obesity is a very recent and unprecedented phenomenon. The rapid rise in obesity initially began in the West (principally in the United States) in the 1970s, in parallel with the type of economic development much longed-for by less fortunate countries. Since then, we have been little more than helpless bystanders of its inexorable march forward, a phenomenon which has proved itself capable of overcoming anything and everything we have tried to put in its way.

Obesity has reached all corners of the globe, all segments of the population and all social classes, and is affecting all age groups, from the elderly down to the youngest, without exception.

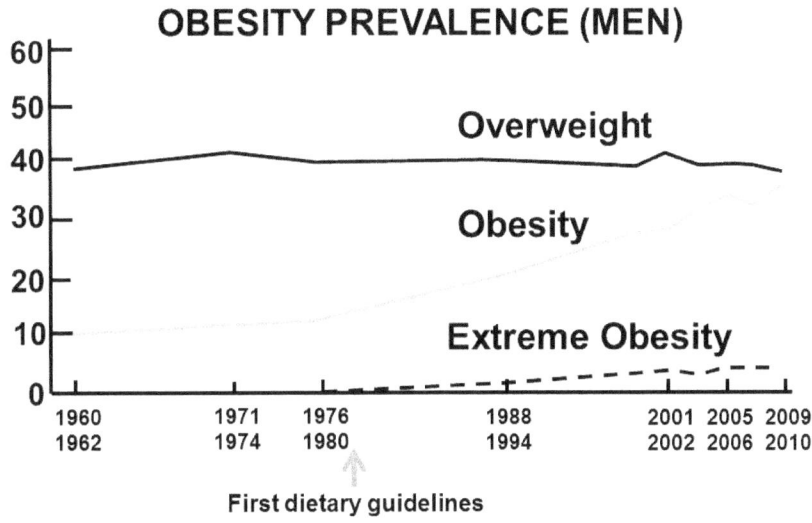

Trend in obesity in the U.S. (data provided by the *Centre for Disease Control*)

For many years, this epidemic of obesity was thought to have a simple solution: if we eat more than we need to, what we need to do to combat obesity is to expend more energy (do more physical exercise) and reduce our calorie intake. As simple as pie... but equally useless. We obviously eat more than we need to and eating less would contribute to solving the problem but, for some reason, we're incapable of doing so; in fact, we're eating more and more. After years of spending huge sums of money on awareness campaigns and nutritional education programmes promoting these recommendations, the net result has been... zero.

What's behind this modern-day obsession with overeating? Could it be, as is commonly suggested in some circles, that we have become gluttonous and idle? Is it all just a question of willpower, or perhaps more correctly, the lack of it? Some would say it's just a matter of taking the right decision (eat less and expend more energy) and sticking to it. In fact, as we shall see in later chapters, many people believe that obese people have less willpower and are incapable of taking and sticking to the decision which is most convenient for them. In short, that it's their fault if they're fat. Once again, however, this idea is prejudiced and totally void of any evidence to support it. Is it really plausible to think that people 20 years ago had more willpower and a greater sense of responsibility?

All these arguments are as simplistic as they are useless. Human nature has not undergone any significant changes in recent times: our genes are the same as they were 30 or 40 years ago and so is our physiology. Conversely, what *has* changed radically is our environment and the food we eat, and it seems clear that this does have an effect not only on our physiology and metabolism but also on our brain, and in a big way. After all, our brain takes the final decision to eat or not to eat.

Leaving aside prejudices and incriminatory arguments, what is beyond dispute is that obese people frequently take a decision to eat which is not based on their energy requirements. Or rather, their brain and neurons, the home of the decision-making process, take this decision. So let's now take a more in-depth look into these issues and the reasons behind them all. Whilst doing so, don't forget the two perspectives on eating that we are already familiar with: on one hand, that associated with energy homeostasis, and on the other, the more hedonic perspective associated with feelings and desires.

2.1. WHEN THE "THERMOSTAT" GOES WRONG

As we saw in the first part of this book, the neurons of the hypothalamus act like switches, triggering the feeling of satiety or of appetite depending on the messages channelled through to them at different stages of the digestive process. These messages are normally generated in the presence of certain hormones and other signals of the digestive system which are detected by the corresponding neuronal receptors.

Though researchers had, until quite recently, only identified a limited number of these hormones, modern-day research in the field of endocrinology is prolific in identifying new peptides which modulate all these signals in one way or another and which in some way impact on the final effect. Given that the presence (or not) of hormones plays such a key role in energy regulation and appetite, it is logical that researchers have spent years studying their behaviour in our body and comparing their concentration levels in normal weight people with that of obese people, particularly immediately after a meal. Results clearly reveal important differences.

Though it's always remarkable to witness how nature manages to ensure balance in the operational functioning of a living being, putting together and coordinating a wide range of different interrelated actions, there are occasions when this complex system does not function as it should. One such case is when it is confronted with obesity.

Let's look at the case of one specific hormone; insulin, which plays a particularly important role as one of the key players in the metabolism of glucose, the most common source of energy our body normally has to deal with.

Carbohydrates and glucose

After we have eaten food which is rich in digestible carbohydrates (for example, bread, cereals, biscuits, rice or pasta), the acids and enzymes of our digestive system progressively break the food down into its most basic component units, mainly glucose molecules. At different stages of the process, these molecules are absorbed into the bloodstream and subsequently transported around the body to be used as a source of energy for muscles and tissues, as well as for our brain.

The metabolism of glucose has been extensively studied due to its key role in energy homeostasis. However, its capacity as an energy provider is not the only reason for our interest in it, as it is also related to certain diseases such as diabetes. Though the presence of glucose in our blood is normal and necessary, its presence in excessively high quantities is, as diabetics know only too well, highly dangerous, as the incapacity to correctly control concentration levels of glucose in the bloodstream is a defining characteristic of diabetes. Chronically high blood glucose levels invariably brings with it a series of health problems and, in extreme cases, may even cause death. To avoid this, evolution has equipped us with a powerful mechanism to maintain these levels under control; a polypeptide known as insulin. Produced by the so-called beta cells in the pancreas, insulin continuously regulates the absorption of glucose from the blood and enables it to be stored in muscles and other tissues, thereby avoiding potentially dangerous levels of concentration.

Insulin is also involved in many physiological processes, some of which are related to energy storage: for example, the synthesis of lipids and the use of fats as an energy source, to mention but one. The point I'm making is that if all the functions of insulin are taken into consideration within the context of that complex concept of energy regulation under discussion here, the principal role of this hormone could be considered to be that of helping our metabolism to properly store and accumulate energy. Furthermore, as well as all these metabolic issues, the brain also uses blood glucose levels as an indicator to manage satiety. The higher the glucose levels, the fuller we should normally feel.

Well, let's take a look at the problems involved. Results from numerous studies have revealed that a large percentage of overweight people present alterations in one part of this theoretical system when compared to thin people. More specifically, overweight people tend to have abnormally high levels of insulin in the blood, especially after meals. This phenomenon is known as hyperinsulinemia and is considered to be one of the key factors in the diagnosis of this metabolic syndrome, one of the most prevalent health problems in modern society. What causes hyperinsulinemia? Are insulin levels high because our blood glucose levels are also too high (for example, after eating a lot of fast-digesting carbohydrates) and the insulin is therefore necessary to correctly manage this situation? Is there a reason for the pancreas malfunctioning and producing excess insulin?

Scientists have identified that excessively high levels of insulin in the blood is often preceded and accompanied by a desensitisation towards insulin itself. It would seem that the receptors responsible for detecting insulin stop functioning as they should and become progressively less effective over time. Consequently, as time passes, more insulin is required to manage the same amount of glucose. This condition is known as insulin resistance. As we shall see in later chapters of this book, the origin of insulin resistance is, as yet, unclear, and is in fact the source of considerable scientific controversy, though consensus has been reached on the idea that it is exacerbated by obesity. Everything would point to the fact that its development can be put down to a series of factors.

From a metabolic perspective, hyperinsulinemia (high levels of insulin in the blood) facilitates fat storage, which is not exactly a favourable scenario when considering how to combat obesity. Moreover, the outlook hardly improves when we analyse the issue from the perspective of appetite and satiety.

I'll explain. Take a good look at the sequence of events under analysis:

1. Fast-digesting carbohydrates are ingested.

2. The food is digested and the carbohydrates pass into the bloodstream in the form of glucose.

3. If your metabolism is insulin resistant, blood insulin levels must be higher than normal and consequently soar (hyperinsulinemia) to be able to manage all the glucose.

4. This excess of insulin eventually gives rise to a sharp fall in glucose.

As mentioned above, high glucose levels trigger the feeling of satiety in the brain. This typically occurs around half an hour after starting a meal. However, around an hour or two later, the counter-effect – the sharp fall in glucose due to the excess of insulin – kicks in, and low glucose levels usually trigger a feeling of being hungry and, with it, that other all-too-familiar feeling for those who are overweight: the craving for more carbohydrates, despite the fact that your stomach still feels full.

At this point, let's look a little deeper into the relation between glucose and the brain, and with a particular focus on the chronic presence of these sharp fluctuations described above. The brain routinely uses glucose as a fuel and can source it in different ways. If your diet is high in carbohydrates, the brain's preferred source of glucose is the bloodstream as it can be found there in abundance. To reach the brain, glucose must first pass through the so-called blood-brain barrier (BBB), which separates the circulatory system from the brain and its fluids. This barrier, the main and crucial function of which is to ensure the brain's surroundings are kept in optimum condition, is very selectively permeable. In this respect, only when a glucose saturation point is reached, i.e. over and above a certain concentration level, does the barrier allow the passage of glucose, which then reaches the neurons by means of a specific biochemical transporter protein known as Glucose Transporter 1 or GLUT1. If the neurons are very active and in need of more fuel, they will send out the corresponding chemical signals to their surrounding environment. More GLUT1 transporter proteins will subsequently be produced to capture more glucose through the blood-brain barrier for its immediate use.

Some mechanism, don't you think? Well, it would be if it always worked like it should do. Sometimes it breaks down or is simply thrown off balance by the presence of insulin resistance. When this happens, the sensitivity of the receptors of this hormone diminishes, causing them not to detect it as they should. As a result, the delicate biochemical balance of the brain to obtain energy from glucose in the quantities required may be affected and malfunction. Or, put in simpler and clearer terms, the processes involved in supplying fuel to the most important organ of our body are altered.

That doesn't sound very good, does it? Well, unfortunately, it doesn't stop there. Experts looking further into the role of insulin in the brain have found that its capacity to influence goes far beyond the management of energy and satiety. Research has revealed that insulin is involved in a significant proportion of the huge amount of processes and metabolic pathways related to neuronal activity, thereby forming part of the intricate network of biochemical activity taking place in this area. Though we still have a lot to learn about this network, what we can deduce at this point in time is that imbalances such as insulin resistance have a negative effect on various points of the network and unsettle a good deal of the mechanisms designed to regulate it.

According to some experts, if this situation becomes chronic and is maintained over several years, it could lead to irreversible brain damage. Studies on the size and structure of the brain, conducted both through autopsies and using non-invasive techniques on living people, have found a relation between the metabolic syndrome – the term used to refer to the presence of obesity, high glucose levels and insulin resistance, high triglycerides, low HDL cholesterol and hypertension – and some serious brain abnormalities such as reduced cognitive capacity and cerebral atrophy (brain shrinkage), even among young people.

But that's not all. Unfortunately, scientists have not only identified imbalances in the management of insulin but in other hormones as well.

Leptin resistance

Leptin, a hormone mainly secreted by our own body fat (fatty tissue) and more directly associated with appetite and satiety than insulin, has aroused great interest among the scientific community ever since it was first discovered relatively recently in 1994. A protein composed of 146 amino acids, leptin is, like all hormones, associated with a large number of control processes in various physiological fields. From a molecular perspective, our fatty tissue produces leptin through the actions of the so-called OB gene. Leptin secretion and concentration are therefore closely correlated to the subcutaneous body fat we have accumulated.

The main attraction of leptin for scientists has been its capacity to regulate appetite: the higher the level of leptin secretion, the greater the reduction in appetite. Leptin levels increase in direct relation to the amount of food we have eaten, and subsequently and progressively diminish when we stop eating. Eventually, low leptin levels also contribute to us feeling hungry again. This behaviour has made leptin especially interesting as a potential tool in the fight against obesity, a field of enormous interest for any researcher.

The explanation as to how leptin suppresses appetite is threefold. Firstly, it activates anorexigenic (POMC) neurons associated with satiety in the hypothalamus. Secondly, it is capable of counteracting certain compounds which activate appetite-inducing AgRP neurons. Thirdly, it favours the synthesis of other compounds capable of inhibiting those neurons. As well as this neutralizing effect on appetite-inducing orexigenic neurons, leptin has another metabolic effect directly related to the possible prevention of obesity: its mere presence is capable of reducing the synthesis of lipids, thereby interfering in the processes related to the creation of fat. Just the opposite of what insulin does.

Though several different leptin receptors (receptors which are leptin-sensitive and trigger the subsequent chain of biochemical and neurological events) have been identified in the area of the hypothalamus, the key player in energy regulation is considered to be the ObRb receptor. Experiments have shown that deficiency of this receptor provokes morbid obesity in animals, thereby giving credence to the hypothesis that the ObRb receptor detects the presence of leptin and activates appetite-inhibiting neurons.

So, as you can see, there are many processes involved in the energy-regulating operations of leptin. Once again, these processes form part of a complex web of interrelations that can be summarised as follows:

1. Food is ingested.

2. Leptin levels rise.

3. Specific receptors detect the presence of leptin.

4. Appetite-inducing neurons are deactivated and appetite-inhibiting neurons are activated.

At this point, you may well be asking yourself the same question as many hopeful researchers were when this hormone was discovered. Which is... if obesity is the consequence of chronic leptin deficiency, couldn't leptin be administered exogenously (externally) to obese people, thereby solving the problem in one fell swoop?

Unfortunately, it's not as easy as that. Far from it. The first obstacle to this solution appeared when evidence arose of something paradoxical and, initially, surprising. Contrary to what could be expected, it was found that most overweight people did not have a low plasma concentration of leptins. In fact, just the opposite: the hormone was found to be present in their blood in higher quantities than normal (hyperleptinemia). Furthermore, attempts to reduce body fat by exogenously administering leptin were unsuccessful. Providing more leptin to suppress appetite failed and, what's more, gave rise to several problems and clinical side effects.

A series of studies conducted at the end of the 1990s shed some light on this issue. Findings revealed that, as is the case with insulin, many obese people suffer from an insensitivity or resistance to leptin. In other words, despite having high blood leptin levels, the leptin itself is not as effective as it should be. In fact, the greater the amount of fatty tissue, the greater leptin resistance would appear to be.

In recent years, since this was discovered, scientists have endeavoured to discover the reasons behind this problem and, at the time of writing, continue to work hard in this area. However, once again, there are no simple, single or definitive answers. The initial hypothesis suggested a possible difficulty for leptin in reaching the brain. Just as in the case of glucose, leptin must first pass through the blood-brain barrier for hypothalamic receptors to detect it and activate or deactivate the corresponding neurons. Though blood leptin levels may be high, cerebrospinal fluid leptin levels in obese people have been found to be relatively low. It would seem that the permeability of the blood-brain barrier is modified for some reason, thereby hindering the passage of the hormone in a sufficiently large quantity to the corresponding area of the brain.

Though many theories have been looked into, experts are now of the opinion that the most likely and the main inducer of this phenomenon is an excess of triglycerides. The role of triglycerides in controlling the blood-brain barrier has been proven, and tests have confirmed that reducing the concentration levels of triglycerides increases the passage of leptin through to cerebrospinal fluid.

The second hypothesis proposed to explain leptin resistance looks more deeply at the signal attenuation of specific leptin receptors, particularly the above-mentioned ObRb receptor, attributable to certain molecular mechanisms. The theory is that the presence of signal inhibitors or suppressors may be hindering the biochemical reactions required for the proper functioning of leptin. More research work than ever is currently being conducted on this hypothesis, analysing the possible habits, processes, reactions and suspect conditions that produce these inhibitors. At the time of writing, liability can most commonly be attributed to:

- an excessive and long-term consumption of fructose and other sugars;

- chronic high levels of insulin; and

- chronic inflammation.

So, it would be fair to say that the situation here is similar to the one we saw in the case of insulin. The existence of leptin resistance prevents this hormone from doing its job properly, throwing the centralised control system of the brain and corresponding specific neurons out of sync. The POMC neurons inducing a feeling of satiety are not activated whilst appetite-inducing AgRP neurons are not deactivated, thereby producing the conditions for feeling hungry even when there is no objective need for energy.

At this point, it should be made clear that, as is the case with other factors related to obesity, there remains a certain amount of controversy regarding leptin resistance as a causal factor of being overweight. Though most experts consider this to be quite likely, the fact that results of many studies point to the reverse, i.e. that obesity itself is a factor which compounds leptin resistance, is not to be overlooked. The most likely explanation is that the two factors feed off each other mutually: in other words, that a certain degree of insensitivity to the hormone increases the likelihood of eating more than is required, and that obesity augments this insensitivity, creating a vicious circle.

It is important to remember that our hormone system is enormously complex, and that all these alterations cannot be exclusively explained by the actions of the two hormones (insulin and leptin) we've looked at to date. Nevertheless, before looking at other imbalances, I'd like to look a little deeper into one of the factors just mentioned as a possible cause of leptin resistance: inflammation.

Inflammation, the silent enemy

Inflammation is a term I'm sure you're familiar with. What's more, I'll be coming back to this word frequently in this book, so I think it's worth learning a little more about it, what it is and how it comes about.

Essentially, inflammation forms part of the biological response of our body tissues to harmful stimuli and injuries such as damaged cells or irritants. The purpose of inflammation is to eliminate the initial cause of cell injury, clear out necrotic cells or tissues and initiate the process of tissue repair. The best-known and most familiar type of inflammation for most of us is acute inflammation, as this is what we see most often when a specific part of our body swells up, turns red and becomes painful. Inflammation comes about through the increased circulation of plasma and leukocytes (white blood cells) from the blood into the injured tissues. A series of biochemical events initiates the inflammatory response, involving the local vascular system, the immune system and cells within the injured tissue. In the early stages of an infection, burn or injury, these cells release compounds which activate the processes that give rise to the clinical symptoms of inflammation. Vasodilation and increased blood flow provoke redness and heat. At the same time, the increased permeability of the blood vessels enables filtration of plasma proteins and the accumulation of fluid (edema) in the tissue, producing a swelling. Some of the compounds released also increase sensitivity to pain.

All these symptoms disappear when the situation returns to normal and the tissue is repaired. When this happens, the damage is considered to have been rectified and the inflammation is believed to have run its course. All of us at some time have been through this type of acute inflammatory process which, at the end of the day, is nothing more than a normal and necessary reaction to replace worn or injured tissue.

The thing is, our organism sometimes reacts this way without any external provocation. No injuries, no pathogens, no visible external attack. However, on a microscopic level, the concentration level of the biocomponents or markers related to the inflammation can be seen to have increased above what can be considered as normal. This is our immune system at work, defending our body. We can't see it and we don't feel it, but it's there.

If this situation recurs regularly, or worse still, if it doesn't disappear or remit over time but becomes continuous, it is considered as chronic inflammation. Unlike acute inflammation, focused on localised tissues, chronic inflammation is characterised by the extensive presence of markers throughout the body, and is therefore often referred to as systemic inflammation. Numerous studies link systemic inflammation to a host of health and disease-related problems, some of which are closely linked to obesity: for example, insulin and leptin resistance, atherosclerosis (obstruction or hardening of the arteries), cardiovascular diseases, high blood pressure and type 2 diabetes, amongst others.

Exactly what causes inflammation is not known for certain, or perhaps it's more accurate to say that many factors are known to cause it. It would seem to be another of those phenomena typical of the developed world, the origin of which can probably be attributed to multiple factors and is difficult to pin down. An excess of certain undesirable foods, a sedentary lifestyle, a high-calorie diet, the consumption of toxic substances (tobacco, alcohol, drugs, etc.), stress... all these factors have been linked to inflammation. Obesity itself perpetuates inflammation; excessive body fat and fat cells would seem to cheat our immune system into mobilising and dispersing its "troops" throughout our body. In people who are considerably overweight, concentration levels of inflammation markers are generally two or three times higher than normal. The following protein types (also referred to as cytokines) are examples of these markers:

- IL-6 (interleukin-6)

- IL-8 (interleukin-8)

- IL-18 (interleukin-18)

- TNF-α (Tumor Necrosis Factor alpha)

- CRP (C-reactive protein)

The presence of these cytokines in our organism also affects our brain and, by extension, the hypothalamus, the area responsible for basic homeostatic control. Findings from recent research have confirmed the presence of several markers of inflammation in this highly sensitive area of the brain related to food intake, and the term "hypothalamic inflammation" has now become part of the clinical vernacular.

By conducting experiments on animals, experts have proved that these inflammatory proteins are capable of interfering in the normal operation of the neurons which regulate our appetite, thereby causing them to become insensitive to certain components and elements considered to be absolutely crucial for energy control. And those components and elements include leptin and insulin, the two hormones we were speaking about just a few pages ago. At least part of the responsibility for the corresponding receptors of these hormones not being able to successfully detect them can probably be laid firmly at the door of chronic inflammation.

Hormones aplenty

After this brief incursion into the concept of chronic or systemic inflammation, let's now return to the subject of hormones, as insulin and leptin are not the only ones linked to obesity. In recent times, other hormones have progressively been discovered which, apart from performing several different biological functions, have been found to be related to energy homeostasis. Around one hundred of them - too many to be listed and discussed here on these pages - are currently the subject of intensive research. Very little is currently known about many of these hormones, though it is likely that the role they have in relation to obesity is very limited. However, some of them do need mentioning, as experts have confirmed their relevance to the subject under discussion in this book.

One of them is ghrelin, an orexigenic hormone, i.e. an appetite stimulant, the opposite of leptin. Discovered towards the end of the 1990s, ghrelin is primarily secreted by cells in different parts of the digestive tract, particularly after stomach emptying. Ghrelin receptors (referred to as GHSR1a) are scattered around different areas of the brain, including those related to appetite. This hormone not only activates the NPY/AgRP orexigenic neurons of the hypothalamus but also those involved in the reward circuit we looked at in the previous section of this book; for example, dopaminergic neurons. In other words, it has a regulatory role in both homeostatic and hedonic eating.

The effect of ghrelin is of particular interest. At high concentration levels, it can amplify the pleasure produced by foods. As a result, even though other hormones may have done their job in creating conditions conducive to feeling full, if ghrelin concentration levels are high, what we actually feel may be very different to what can be expected. This same phenomenon may exaggerate our expectations of the pleasure that eating a particular food will give us, thereby driving us to crave it and causing us to focus all our efforts on getting our hands on it.

Stress, depression and insufficient sleep are all, unfortunately, characteristic features of modern-day life. Of more concern, however, is the fact that they have been linked to high levels of ghrelin in the bloodstream. Studies have revealed that a negative mentality or guilty feeling when eating (for example, thinking that something is particularly fattening) impedes the reduction of ghrelin levels after a meal, probably because of the anguish and stress this idea triggers in us.

Elementary logic would lead us to think that, as well as all the other variables that make things difficult for them, obese people would have high levels of ghrelin in their bloodstream. Not true. In fact, as with leptin, it's just the opposite. Once again, it would seem we are faced with a situation of insensitivity or resistance, a scenario in which the corresponding neurons struggle to react to the presence of this hormone. If this is so, this situation may impact on the reward circuit, or more specifically on the activity of dopamine, altering the way it and its receptors work and triggering behaviour related to a higher intake of food. And that, for the moment, is as much as I can say about this. Ghrelin is involved in a complex network of interactions with other biocomponents. At the time of writing, the origin and implications of this insensitivity and its relation to eating habits and food constituents are the subject of considerable research, with various hypotheses being put forward.

Whatever, ghrelin is not the only hormone secreted by the gastrointestinal system. There are many others connected to food intake and appetite, often less directly and in some cases performing a regulatory rule on other hormones and components. For example, GLP-1 is a gastrointestinal peptide hormone mainly secreted in the small intestine which stimulates the release of insulin in the pancreas and inhibits glucagon, thereby combating the phenomenon of insulin resistance discussed earlier in this chapter and bringing about a rapid reduction in blood glucose levels. For this very reason, GLP-1 is used in medication for type 2 diabetes sufferers. Peptide YY (PYY) is a component secreted in the intestine and known to have an inhibiting effect on appetite and stomach emptying. PYY concentration levels fall prior to eating and increase immediately after eating, so the fact that blood PYY levels in overweight people are often low could be an influential factor on their condition. Cholecystokinin (CCK) is a hormone principally secreted in the small intestine which, as well as releasing various digestive enzymes, acts as an appetite suppressant on interacting with orexigenic neurons.

And the list goes on. These are just a few of the best-known and most studied hormones involved in the system with which our brain and our intestine are in constant dialogue to modulate, amongst other things, energy flow and food intake. This incredible and complex mind-stomach dialogue is conducted through nerve channels running throughout our body, most of which are ramifications of the vagus nerve, one of the main bundles of communication "cables" in the human body. The vagus nerve starts at the brain stem and runs through to the digestive system via the body's major organs (heart, lungs, etc.).

The nerve endings which reach our intestine are equipped with receptors which react to the presence of all these hormones and, consequently, generate and relay signals through our body to the brain. These signals are then processed on the basis of a huge amount of other filtered information coming into the brain via other channels, and especially taking into consideration the signals being detected by the brain neurons themselves in their own particular environment, both those of the hypothalamus and those forming part of the reward circuit. If you remember the numbers involved when we spoke about the principles of how the brain operates in the first part of this book, then you will further appreciate just how incredibly complex this dialogue is.

In short, the list of obesity-related hormones is long and continues to grow. For decades, attempts were made to establish direct relations between these hormones and obesity, but scientific research is now showing that it's not as simple as that. A hormone may play a direct role in a particular biochemical or metabolic process but also, due to its impact on other variables, an indirect role in others. The outcome of all this is a tangled web of interactions which is very difficult to unravel. However, within this web, these hormones play the role of key supporting actors in regulating food intake and energy homeostasis, and all this in clear synergy with the leading actor: the brain. We know that hormone synthesis depends on a number of factors, one of the most important of which is neuronal activity, so we can deduce that the brain, that powerful central processor, is not only influenced by hormones but also regulates them, giving orders to secrete them in greater or lesser quantities.

The conclusion could be drawn that what scientific evidence is showing us is that when obesity is present, this web or network undergoes a profound change due to various factors, some of which are still unknown to us. Certain symptoms, such as the afore-mentioned resistance to some of these hormones, give us an insight into where we should continue researching, but all these hypotheses converge in the need for further in-depth research into one common factor: the relation between the brain and the digestive system.

A microworld inside us

Having focused so much on the cerebral side of this issue, and despite the fact that we are continuously speaking about obesity and eating, not much has been said so far about our digestive system. As we've just seen, a considerable number of hormones are secreted there so this is by no means an issue to be ignored. In fact, though the main players here will continue to be neurons, I'd like briefly to digress and focus on one particular part of our digestive system; the intestine. Until recently, this organ did not generally arouse much interest in the general population, but it is now the subject of a lot more discussion. And there's good reason for this to continue being the case.

Most of us know that the intestine is the tract through which food components are absorbed, via the intestinal walls, into the bloodstream, and where food finishes its journey through our digestive system as excrement. However, what we don't perhaps know is just how special this organ is when observed under a microscope. The intestine is home to billions of microorganisms of around one thousand different species. The most abundant of these microorganisms are bacteroidetes, firmicutes and actinobacteria. All this microscopic life form is what we used to call *intestinal flora*; nowadays, this is more correctly referred to as *microbiota* or the *microbiome*, as these microorganisms are neither plants nor flowers.

The intestine is not the only place in our body where large numbers of bacteria live in harmony with us. This same situation of symbiosis is also present in other parts of the body, such as the vagina. However, in this case, intestinal microbes play a key role in the final stage of food processing and absorption. These microscopic living beings are instrumental in the metabolisation of nutrients and perform other very important activities. For example, their presence serves to protect us from the colonisation of other potentially harmful microorganisms, thereby acting as an immune defence mechanism. They also have a significant role to play in the mucous membrane lining the inner wall of the intestine, which modulates the absorption of food. This is a key stage of digestion, when the nutrients pass from the digestive system into our bloodstream, permeating the intestinal walls to be distributed around the body in our blood. The state and composition of the mucosa, including its microbial composition, are factors which contribute greatly to the process of correct absorption in line with our relevant physiological requirements.

Where does this relatively new interest in the relationship between microbiota and obesity come from? In recent years, findings from numerous studies have identified important differences between the microbial colonies in obese people and in normal weight people. There would seem to be a clear link between being overweight and certain significant alterations in the type and quantity of intestinal microbes. This imbalance normally takes the form of a shortage of bacteria which could be considered as beneficial, and an excess of harmful bacteria which may produce undesirable effects for our organism. It must also be said at this point that the findings from these studies are mixed; not all of them have reached this same conclusion. What's more, most of them are observational studies, a fact which always raises doubts over how causality has been determined.

However, another type of test conducted on mice, in which their microbiota is modified at will (in some cases, even leaving them without any), would seem to provide prima facie evidence that an imbalance in the distribution of microbial species may have an impact on health problems and excess weight. If the microbiota of an obese mouse is transplanted into a thin mouse, the latter has been seen to gain weight. Furthermore, it has also been proved that people's intestinal microbiota changes when their diet is modified, though we still don't know exactly to what extent, what specifically causes this and the exact correlations involved (what foodstuff or nutrient affects what species of microorganism).

There are certain specific situations for which experts propose quite detailed and clear-cut hypotheses and mechanisms. For example, going back to food absorption, it is known that certain bacteria are capable of increasing the permeability of the intestinal wall; as a result, the excess presence of these bacteria may favour the absorption of certain undesirable biocomponents. Why undesirable? Because some of them may interfere in certain metabolic processes and be linked to chronic inflammation. These intruders may also affect the change in the concentration levels of certain hormones, and even their loss of sensitivity towards others. And yes, I'm once again referring to insulin and leptin resistance.

Do you remember that dialogue we spoke of a few pages ago between the gut and the brain? Well, it's not difficult to imagine that an alteration in the microbiota state would likely distort that conversation in a big way. In fact, it could be concluded that problems in the microbiota could lead to a deterioration in the biochemical balance of our organism, exacerbating inflammation and upsetting hormone concentration levels, thereby affecting neuronal response to incoming signals. And don't forget! When neurons are affected, our own behaviour may also be affected, as they are the cells that make up our brain and which are instrumental in all our decision-making processes.

Screening impairment in the brain

After this short incursion into the intestine, let's now return to brain imbalance. All these issues we are looking at would be much easier to investigate if we could see, in real time and in detail, how the brain actually works, just as a mechanic gets a lot of information by simply looking at an engine in disrepair when it's running. Unfortunately, however, the brain is not a big engine made up of a few hundred pieces, and neuronal activity is microscopic.

Irrespective of this, it's an exciting challenge. Researchers have been working towards this goal for years and have made spectacular progress. Modern brain imaging techniques are the result of constructive collaboration between different scientific disciplines, medicine, physics and engineering, and have enabled one of neuroscientists' greatest wishes to come true: to be able to observe each area of the brain in isolation and in action. Previously, they had had to make do with an electroencephalogram (EEG), which enabled them to comprehensively monitor all the small electric signals being generated under our cranium, at different frequencies and wavelengths, but only capable of providing them with limited information. Fortunately, neuroscientists discovered that when an area of the brain is especially active, it undergoes physical and physiological changes that can be detected. To be exact, the arterial and venous vessels dilate, triggering a greater inflow of oxygen and reducing the relative quantity of a molecule called deoxyhemoglobin (formed as a consequence of oxyhemoglobin releasing its oxygen to the tissues). The polar or magnetic nature of deoxyhemoglobin enables differences in its concentration levels to be detected by certain sensors.

The knowledge gained from these discoveries has enabled us to go far beyond what was previously possible, to the point of now being able to generate a graphic and visual representation of brain activity. This technology, known as Functional Magnetic Resonance Imaging (fMRI), is of enormous use and value in many medical activities, and is particularly valuable in helping neurosurgeons to plan their operations and to avoid – or at least minimise – possible damage to the brain that may be caused by having to remove or slice into one of its parts.

Given the enormous importance of the brain in processes related to food and eating, scientists have also begun to use fMRI as a research tool into obesity. In turn, this has enabled them to confirm that when it comes to eating, brain activity, both prior to and after food intake, is more complex than was initially thought decades ago, involving areas of the brain far beyond the hypothalamus and overlapping with the reward areas described in a previous chapter of this book.

I should like to emphasize that research using this technology is in full swing and has really only just started, so it's likely that the conclusions and hypotheses currently being taken forward on the basis of fMRI will be considerably expanded. I therefore recommend that you bear this in mind while reading the paragraphs immediately below.

One of the most repeated experiments using fMRI has been to observe brain activity prior to food intake. Through these experiments, it has been found that the brains of obese people do not react in the same way as those of normal weight people. More specifically, it has been seen that the areas which are activated (by visual images, smells, thoughts, etc.) prior to eating – those which make a food appetising for us, which generate expectation and give us the urge to eat it – are more keenly stimulated among obese people. And as a result, these people feel a greater desire and incentive to go looking for food. Do you remember when we spoke about the capacity of dopaminergic neurons to generate expectation? Well, here it is.

In practice, the outcome is that this behaviour is normally (and unfortunately) interpreted as a lack of willpower. The truth, as we have seen in previous chapters of this book, is that the neural response of this type of people to certain stimuli is in some way exaggerated, complicating inhibition and preparing and mobilising their organism for one specific action: eating.

Another area of research typical in this field is to observe what happens next, i.e. at the intake stage, to study the effect that the actual fact of starting to eat has on neuronal activity. Once again, it has been found that many areas of the brain are involved, including the reward areas, and that the results vary depending on the degree to which the subjects under study are overweight. In this case, the reverse was found, i.e. that the activity in the reward areas amongst obese people is lower than that in normal weight people, seemingly tempered and reflecting a limited or reduced sense of pleasure. This could be interpreted as "an unsatisfactory meal".

In short, the possibility of seeing the brain in operation has enabled us to identify that something changes or is altered internally when a person is overweight. The brain is activated more than it normally would be just by the sight of food, but actually eating that food activates it less than can be expected. Please remember this circumstance... it's going to take on particular importance in future chapters.

The biological clock

For now, though not for very long, let's leave fMRI and neurological screening to one side and continue our look at other possible imbalances of the brain related to obesity. More specifically, let's take a look at one of the great mysteries: the process of sleeping, the absolutely essential need to sleep. The moment when the body of all animals with a brain seems to disconnect and enter into a kind of strange coma.

Actually, this would be a terrifying state of affairs if we didn't know beforehand what was going on. Whilst our muscles and senses become, to all intents and purposes, sidelined, our brain continues to be very active, operating in a surprisingly autonomous way, playing around with our consciousness and isolated from any type of external stimulus. The exact reason why we need to sleep remains a mystery for science. In theory, for the brain to be operative without the body exerting any type of "conscious" control over it for several hours is, in evolutionary terms, highly unfavourable. While this process is in course, a living being is totally defenceless and at the mercy of any predator. Nevertheless, and without exception in nature, all animals with a brain need to sleep: some more, others less, and in different ways, and it would seem we have no alternative other than to continue doing so, as the effects of sleep deprivation are well-known and have been so for many years. In extreme cases, or when we are forced to remain awake for several days, the severe problems and psychological and neurological disorders this causes are clearly visible: general and deep-rooted malaise, memory problems, behavioural disorders and even a deterioration in mental health. Acute sleep deprivation may even cause death, as in those cases, fortunately few and far between, of severe neurological illnesses which prevent the patient from sleeping.

The human sleep-wake cycle, as is the case for most higher animals, is, for obvious reasons, closely linked to basic astronomy and the day-night cycle created by the relationship between the Earth and the Sun. As human beings, we have evolved in an environment in which we have adapted to being active and conscious during the day, in sunlight hours, and to "disconnecting" at night, when it's dark. The duration of this cycle is around 24 hours. These biological variations, synchronised mainly (though not exclusively) with sunlight, are known as circadian rhythms, and are reliable harbingers of certain cyclical and physiological changes (principally hormone-modulated) seen in living creatures. And sleep is one of those changes.

Sleep has probably gone hand-in-hand with living creatures for many millions of years. Scientists have found evidence of basic sleep mechanisms in small worm-like creatures known to have existed on the face of the Earth many years ago (there are signs of their presence 700 million years ago). These creatures exhibit melatonin production cycles in their organism synchronised with natural light. The same thing happens in our brain; melatonin is a hormone involved in the package of biochemical changes that trigger our need to sleep and which maintain our brain in the required state for the required amount of time.

However, though we may be able to surmise the reasons behind the scope and duration of these cycles, a biological and biochemical explanation for the need to sleep has proved elusive to scientists... until very recently. New research seems to have thrown some light on this scientific darkness. The most widely-accepted hypotheses drawn from the latest studies in this area suggest that sleep may be a state in which many activities and important physiological and neurological tasks are performed, but that primarily, it is the time used by our organism for eliminating waste from the brain. As we know, neuronal activity is the product of a complex network of biochemical reactions which, like all reactions of this type, produce other products and sub-products as waste. These waste products are deposited in the interstitial fluid around the previously active neurons. If concentration levels of this waste are excessively high, it may interfere in subsequent processes, hindering the necessary reactions and bringing about neurological alterations and symptoms of alarm. Just as our lymphatic system takes charge of removing waste from the rest of our body, it would appear there is another system in the brain, already baptised by some as the *glymphatic system*, that performs this same function. This system, therefore, would be composed of cerebrospinal fluid (a transparent liquid that bathes the brain and spinal cord) mixed with the liquid that bathes the neurons (the interstitial liquid), flushing out unwanted metabolites from the organ.

In truth, the brain maintains a constant cleansing process, not just while we are asleep. However, it would seem that while the brain is active, it is not capable of managing all the waste which is being produced. During sleep, "normal" activity is considerably reduced and certain environment variables may change, as has been confirmed through observing the brains of animals at sleep. Experts have found that the flow of cerebrospinal fluid increases, as does the interstitial space, whilst certain metabolites are removed much more quickly than usual and concentration levels of certain waste products diminish rapidly. Without this process (in other words, if we don't sleep), waste accumulates and interferes with neuronal activity, particularly in synapses, giving rise to the acute symptoms mentioned above.

If this hypothesis were correct, it would logically pose the question of whether a significant (though not acute) reduction in the amount of sleep could affect the effectiveness of these waste management processes and, as a result, of how the brain operates, especially if this becomes chronic and is maintained over long periods of time. Or if our sleep-wake rhythm is constantly broken up by continuous changes in lifestyle habits (shift work, travelling frequently, etc.), thereby disrupting the processes.

Well, it seems that this, effectively, is the case. Many observational studies link a lack of sleep to being overweight and many other health problems. Furthermore, many intervention trials have shown how a person's metabolism changes significantly under these conditions. For example, if a person is following a hypocaloric diet, it has been established that insufficient sleep makes it difficult to lose weight. At the same time, cortisol levels go up considerably, potentially interfering in other metabolic processes as we shall see a little later. Moreover, indicators related to the metabolism of glucose and carbohydrates, used to predict insulin resistance and possible type-2 diabetes, are negatively affected, ghrelin (an appetite stimulating hormone) levels increase and leptin (a hunger inhibiting hormone) levels decline. In these cases, a greater appetite at night and a heightened preference for highly palatable foods is often observed. Some genetic tests conducted on twins even suggest that certain genes linked to a predisposition to obesity may be activated or expressed more easily, and that people who sleep less have shorter telomeres (buffers at the end of chromosomes), associated with a shorter life expectancy.

In any case, and as mentioned above, light is the main signal our brain uses to modulate circadian rhythms. Our exposure to light, including sunlight, has changed radically in recent decades, to the point where we're hardly ever without it. If we add the disruption of sleep patterns to a lack of restful sleep (thereby triggering possible problems of waste removal around neurons), it's not unreasonable to conclude that our brain could consequently be suffering from minor imbalances affecting its capacity to control the whole of our metabolism.

REFERENCES

Return of hunger following a relatively high carbohydrate breakfast is associated with earlier recorded glucose peak and nadir (Chandler-Laney et al, 2014)

Lipolytic suppression following carbohydrate ingestion limits fat oxidation during exercise. (Horowitz et al, 1997)

Metabolic response to carbohydrate ingestion during exercise in males and females. (Wallis et al, 2006)

Cerebral damage in obesity associated metabolic syndrome (Rusinek et al, 2014)

Is your brain to blame for weight regain? (Cornier, 2011)

Insulin Action in Brain Regulates Systemic Metabolism and Brain Function (Kleinridders et al, 2014)

Banting Lecture 2011; Hyperinsulinemia: Cause or Consequence? (2012)

Hyperinsulinemia: A unifying theory of chronic disease? (2015)

Insulin resistance is a cellular antioxidant defense mechanism (2009)

Insulin resistance protects the heart from fuel overload in dysregulated metabolic states (2013)

Insulin resistance as a physiological defense against metabolic stress: implications for the management of subsets of type 2 diabetes (2013)

Impaired insulin action in the human brain: causes and metabolic consequences (2015)

Higher glucose levels associated with lower memory and reduced hippocampal microstructure (Kerti, 2013)

Sensoty.specific appetition: Postingestive detection of glucose rapidly promotes continued consumption of recently encountered flavor (Myers et al, 2012)

20 years of leptin: Connecting leptin signaling to biological function (Allison et al, 2014)

Leptin activates anorexigenic POMC neurons through a neural network in the arcuate nucleus (Cowley et al, 2001)

Advances in understanding the interrelations between leptin resistance and obesity (Pan et al, 2014)

Dietary components in the development of leptin resistance (Vaselli et al, 2013)

Leptin resistance and the response to positive energy balance (Morrison, 2008)

Leptin resistance: a prediposing factor for diet-induced obesity (Scarpace et al, 2009)

Diet-induced obesity leads to the development of leptin resistance in vagal afferent neurons (Lartigue et al, 2011)

The blood-brain barrier as a cause of obesity (Banks et al, 2008)

Triglycerides induce leptin resistance at the blood-brain barrier (Banks et al, 2004)

Triglyceride sensing in the reward circuitry: A new insight in feeding behaviour regulation (Cansell et al, 2015)

Does Hypothalamic Inflammation Cause Obesity? (Wissé y oros, 2009)

Hypothalamic damage is associated with inflammatory markers and worse cognitive performance in obese subjects (Puig et al, 2014)

Bacteria, viruses, and hypothalamic inflammation: Potential new players in obesity (Wierucka-Rybak et al, 2014)

Hypothalamic inflammation and the central nervous system control of energy homeostasis (Pimentel et al, 2014)

Hypothalamic inflammation in the control of metabolic function (Valdearcos et al, 2015)

Ghrelin signalling and obesity: At the interface of stress, mood and food reward (Schellekens et al, 2012)

Diet-induced obesity causes ghrelin resistance in arcuate NPY/AgRP neurons (Briggs et al, 2010)

Metabolic status regulates ghrelin function on energy homeostasis (Briggs et al, 2011)

Ghrelin-mediated appetite regulation in the central nervous system (Kirsz et al, 2011)

Ghrelin mimics fasting to enhance human hedonic, orbitofrontal cortex, and hippocampal responses to food (Goldstone et al, 2014)

Ghrelin enhances cue-induced bar pressing for high fat food (2015)

Mind over milkshakes: mindsets, not just nutrients, determine ghrelin response (Crum et al, 2011)

The future role of gut hormones in the treatment of obesity (Troke et al, 2014

Effects of meals high in carbohydrate, protein, and fat on ghrelin and peptide YY secretion in prepubertal children (Lomenick et al, 2009

High protein intake stimulates postprandial GLP1 and PYY release (van der Klaauw AA et al, 2011)

Comparison of postprandial profiles of ghrelin, active GLP-1, and total PYY to meals varying in fat and carbohydrate and their association with hunger and the phases of satiety (Gibbons et al, 2013)

Gastrointestinal hormones and the dialogue between gut and brain (Dockray, 2014)

Obesity, inflammation, and the gut microbiota (Cox et al, 2014)

Microbiome: A complicated relationship status (Deweerdt, 2014)

The Gut Microbiota Reduces Leptin Sensitivity and the Expression of the Obesity-Suppressing Neuropeptides Proglucagon (Gcg) and Brain-Derived Neurotrophic Factor (Bdnf) in the Central Nervous System (Schele et al, 2013)

The Role of Gut Microbiota on Insulin Resistance (Caricilli et al, 2013)

Meta-analyses of human gut microbes associated with obesity and IBD (Walters y otros 2014)

The Influence of Whole Grain Products and Red Meat on Intestinal Microbiota Composition in Normal Weight Adults: A Randomized Crossover Intervention Trial (2014)

Microbes on the mind (Shen, 2015)

Neuroimaging and obesity: current knowledge and future directions. (Carnell S et al, 2012)

Reward processing in obesity, substance addiction and non-substance addiction (García et al, 2014)

Obesity, Food, and Addiction: Emerging Neuroscience and Clinical and Public Health Implications (Potenza, 2013)

Relation of obesity to consummatory and anticipatory food reward (Stice et al, 2013)

Abdominal fat is associated with a greater brain reward response to high-calorie food cues in Hispanic women. (Luo S et al, 2013)

Emotional eating is associated with increased brain responses to food-cues and reduced sensitivity to GLP-1 receptor activation (Biomendaa et al, 2015)

Relative ability of fat and sugar tastes to activate reward, gustatory, and somatosensory regions. (Stice E et al, 2013)

Gastroenteric hormone responses to hedonic eating in healthy humans (Monteleone et al, 2013)

Melatonin Signaling Controls Circadian Swimming Behavior in Marine Zooplankton - (Tosches, 2014)

Sleep duration and obesity among adults: a meta-analysis of prospective studies (Wu et al, 2014)

Sleep Drives Metabolite Clearance from the Adult Brain (Xie et al, 2013)

Sleep Restriction Enhances the Daily Rhythm of Circulating Levels of Endocannabinoid 2-arachidonoylglycerol (2015)

Insufficient sleep undermines dietary efforts to reduce adiposity (Nedeltcheva et al, 2010)

Metabolic and endocrine effects of sleep deprivation (Copinschi, 2005)

Sub-chronic sleep restriction causes tissue specific insulin resistance (Madhu et al, 2014)

Sleep restriction for 1 week reduces insulin sensitivity in healthy men (Buxton et al, 2010)

Meta-Analysis of Short Sleep Duration and Obesity in Children and Adults (Capuccio et al, 2008)

Sleep duration and body mass index in twins: a gene-environment interaction (Watson et al, 2012)

Dietary intake following experimentally restricted sleep in adolescents (Beebe et al, 2013)

Acute Sleep Deprivation Enhances the Brain's Response to Hedonic Food Stimuli: An fMRI Study (Benedict et al, 2012)

Sleep restriction leads to increased activation of brain regions sensitive to food stimuli (St-Onge et al, 2012)

Increased impulsivity in response to food cues after sleep loss in healthy young men (Cedernaes et al, 2015)

The Internal Circadian Clock Increases Hunger and Appetite in the Evening Independent of Food Intake and Other Behaviors (Scheer et al, 2013)

Sleep Restriction Enhances the Daily Rhythm of Circulating Levels of Endocannabinoid 2-arachidonoylglycerol (2015)

Circadian regulation of metabolism (Bailey et al, 2014)

Meta-analysis on night shift work and risk of metabolic syndrome (wang et al, 2014)

Acute dim light at night increases body mass, alters metabolism, and shifts core body temperature circadian rhythms (Borniger et al, 2014)

Light as a central modulator of circadian rhythms, sleep and affect (LeGates et al, 2014)

2.2. EMOTIONS AND ADDICTIONS

So far in this book, we've spoken about food and eating, and about our metabolism and its relation with the brain, in a rather rational, aseptic and, perhaps, even cold or detached way. The sciences of biochemistry and neurology have established the framework within which we have progressed so far, and as with all scientific disciplines, the bottom line has been rigour and objectivity.

However, when the brain and food are spoken about in the same breath, then emotions, feelings and the more subjective perspective of being overweight inevitably enter the conversation. Why? Because it's obvious that, for us human beings, eating is much more than a mere physiological need, a purely metabolic act or simply a hypothalamic-controlled process.

In this respect, though all of us readily associate the term "emotion" with many different concepts and interpretations, the conceptualisation of this from a scientific perspective is much more complicated. We're very clear about the fact that emotion originates in the brain, despite the fact that, throughout history, different cultures have believed our emotions originate in different areas or components of our body (our blood, our heart, our guts, etc.). Neurologists and psychiatrists have been able to compile a detailed breakdown of the different areas of the brain where emotions are aroused, and many of the biochemical mechanisms involved: sadness, joy, anguish, fear... all of them are brought about by the activity of specific groups of neurons activated by different types of neurotransmitters. Though many people would not be happy with such a non-abstract perspective on the subject, the depth of human feelings would actually seem to be rooted in the earthly, the consequence of the wonderful biochemical twinkling of neurons.

Whatever. For now, let's leave to one side the issue of the feelings that make us want to eat. We'll return to this in more detail later, and in any case, as an introduction, let's first turn our attention to one specific aspect of the relation between emotions and food: the emotional impact of obesity, a kind of negative sentiment associated with being overweight and an issue deserving particular attention.

The stigma of being fat

I don't think a survey has ever been conducted on this question but if obese people were granted three wishes by an imaginary genie of the lamp, for most of them, one of those wishes would undoubtedly be to say goodbye to their obesity.

Though it's not something sufferers would normally or readily own up to, being fat is one of the main reasons behind personal unhappiness. Not so much because it's bad for your health – everyone knows that – but more because of the way it makes you look and the message your appearance conveys to others. Being fat has become a powerful social stigma, one which appears to be spreading at the same unstoppable rate as the increase itself in the prevalence of obesity. This is not a hypothesis based on unsound assumptions or complaints: on the contrary, researchers have been conducting in-depth scientific studies on this issue for several decades. Psychologists have repeatedly and systematically looked into the feelings and the perception that society has of overweight people, regardless of the relationship we may or may not have with them (i.e. as workmates, relatives, friends or strangers). And the findings make for painful reading.

Firstly, on an aesthetic and sexual level, bodies with higher percentages of body fat and which do not conform to fashion standards are rejected out of hand. Whether we like it or not, we are driven by a powerful instinct to choose a physically attractive sexual partner. Furthermore, what is considered as physically attractive is measured against a standard model which, though inaccessible for, and exclusive to, the vast majority of the population, is constantly marketed as the paradigm of health and beauty. Although the members of our species have always made an effort to appear attractive to the opposite sex, as is the case with any species that reproduces sexually, this is probably the first time in history that most of the members of our species consider that objective to be practically beyond their reach. In other words, never before have levels of self-esteem related to self-image been so low. If you are obese, I'm sure you know that painful feeling of "not feeling very attractive", so I don't think I need say any more.

What's more, the problem goes beyond simple unfair and biased comparisons with idealised models which make us feel unhappy and unwanted. Unfortunately, society has developed a strong sense of prejudice towards obese people, a prejudice associated with different aspects of their supposed personality and related to their personal capabilities and worth. And a prejudice which has given rise to covert, cruel and rampant discrimination.

This, sadly, is no exaggeration. Study findings clearly reveal that most of us believe obese people to have less willpower, to be lazier than average and, of course, to be gluttons, the very reason why they are overweight. Why do we think this? Because most of us consider that obese people mostly have only got themselves to blame. And as if that wasn't bad enough, we project these supposed character weaknesses onto other personality traits, leading us to believe obese people are less effective and efficient in their activities, that they are less productive at work and even that they are less intelligent.

Allow me, if you will, to be less politically correct and to make my point loud and clear: most of society considers obese people to be inferior, and even harbours prejudices very similar to those associated with racism or sexism, both of which have been combated vehemently for the last few centuries. I repeat, I am not exaggerating. Data and research on the subject confirm this time and time again. Despite having the same levels of knowledge and competence as thin people, obese people are valued less in all stages and situations of life, from their marks at school through to posts of responsibility in companies.

I imagine you're thinking that these comments are a little sensationalist and that you perhaps can't relate to what I'm saying. You don't discriminate against fat people, do you? Well, we're not normally aware of these prejudices and tend to flatly deny them, systematically fooling ourselves completely. Study findings are quite conclusive and convergent on this issue. This is a fact, and no age or social class is exempt from it. Furthermore, this stigma, potentially related to an increased risk of suffering psychological and personality disorders, remains for life, even if that person manages to slim down at some point in their life. In other words, it's forever.

Perhaps a few detailed examples may help you become more aware of this disturbing reality. All public celebrities who are overweight frequently have to put up with jokes made in bad taste and obnoxious attacks against their physical appearance. Every now and then we hear or read of the unpleasant consequences suffered by people in the public eye (presenters, singers, actors, etc.) who find themselves continually having to explain away their "condition". In this respect, politics is no exception: experts in political marketing are well aware that obesity is a major problem when attempting to gain popularity and votes.

But you don't have to be famous or well-known for people to think you are less capable because you are obese. This prejudice has been seen to be universal, applicable to just about anyone, whatever the relationship between the two parties involved. And we're all guilty of this, even healthcare professionals, the people who should be most aware and sensitive to this issue. For example, normal weight doctors clearly discriminate against their overweight colleagues, considering them to be not so good at their job and believing that patients have less faith in the advice given by them. This belief is confirmed by patients themselves, who generally consider overweight doctors to be less trustworthy and tend to take less notice of their advice and recommendations.

And there's more. This is a two-way phenomenon affecting doctors' attitudes towards patients, to such an extent that it may even have a negative influence on their medical practice. Some research has shown that a high percentage of healthcare professionals dealing with obesity, such as doctors and nutritionists, have a disparaging attitude towards their patients and blame them for being overweight. This would be unthinkable in relation to any other ailment or illness. Such clearly biased attitudes against obese people have even been identified in student practitioners. Of course, this is not something they would openly admit. Just the opposite, in fact: they would probably flatly deny it if they were asked, but by asking the right questions in the right way to ensure they obtain honest and reliable information, it's not been difficult for psychologists to identify this behaviour.

Though the stigma of obesity is hard for anyone to bear, it's especially painful for children and adolescents. Study findings show that the obesity rate among children is increasing in parallel with the increase in obesity itself. What overweight children have to suffer due to their physical and health limitations is compounded by the prejudice they are subjected to by their peers, who, as previously mentioned, usually consider that their obese companions are themselves mostly to blame for their condition. As children have fewer inhibitions than adults, they express these prejudices far more explicitly, thereby creating barriers to friendship and increasing the sense of rejection and isolation in the obese child affected. In some cases, this may even turn into bullying and/or physical and psychological violence which, in turn, can lead to very serious emotional consequences which may haunt victims for the rest of their lives.

In more modern societies, a great effort is made to eradicate any type of discrimination and to promote equal opportunity. However, in contrast with the considerable progress made in combating racism and sexism, hardly any support is available for overweight people. In fact, this stigma is occasionally furthered and consolidated by the very people who are supposedly working to combat it. With the only objective of gaining notoriety, incompetent politicians and publicists serve up disgraceful anti-obesity publicity campaigns to attract attention and maximise their viral marketing, using striking, hard-hitting and stigmatizing messages and images whilst unscrupulously portraying obese people and their families as being mainly to blame for their predicament. And all this despite the fact that study findings have shown time and time again that this type of shock and blame-placing strategy fails to motivate those principally affected to change their habits and to lose weight. Not a year goes by without some country or another mistakenly launching a campaign of this type.

At the risk of sounding repetitive, and just in case there's anyone out there who's still not so sure of what I'm saying, I'd like to finish this chapter by reminding you that not even the best designed and most thorough research studies have managed to prove that obesity is a direct consequence of laziness or a lack of willpower. So, it's high time a serious effort was made to eradicate the unfair stigma attached to obesity, not only on ethical and moral grounds but also because its existence is clearly counterproductive and makes things even more difficult in the battle against being overweight.

Food as a drug

After this initial incursion into the emotional arena and the stigma attached to obesity, let's once again focus our attention on the process of eating and on what this act triggers in our brain. More specifically, let's once again dip into the field of pleasure and reward.

As we've just seen, obesity has an all-round and strongly negative emotional effect on the lives of those who suffer from this condition. However, we've also seen in previous chapters of this book that food can be the source of very positive and rewarding feelings, especially if it comes with certain sensory characteristics designed to provoke a powerful impact on your reward circuit. Just imagine yourself enjoying your favourite food and the wonderful feeling that gives you.

Unfortunately, these perceptions of pleasantness may deteriorate and give way to particularly unpleasant types of behaviour and circumstances. Non-stop eating, struggling to feel full, thinking all the time about food, an intense craving for certain foods (perhaps even at any time of day) and subsequent feelings of guilt… many obese people are probably familiar with at least one or more of these situations. The truth is that many people suffering from excess weight describe their relationship with food in these terms, thereby conveying a certain lack of control over the situation and a complete inability to take charge of this relationship. This type of language is very similar to that used by smokers or alcoholics, or even by those who are addicted to other more toxic and harmful substances which provoke similar behaviour. Or at least, that's what some people who live with this type of behaviour every day tell us.

So, can you become addicted to food? Can a certain food be considered as an addictive substance? Does it make scientific sense to use that type of analogy or comparison? These ideas have gained increasing relevance in recent years, as has the number of exploratory and analytical studies published on the subject. As a result, there is now a considerable body of experts who are of the opinion that one of the potential factors behind the worldwide epidemic of obesity is the capacity of certain foods to become addictive, in a similar way to drugs. Although this approach has its advocates and its opponents, it has given rise to a vast amount of research with very interesting results, which we shall be analysing over the next few pages.

To begin with, let's try to define exactly what we're talking about when we use the term "addiction". In a general sense, it could be said that addiction is a state characterised by the compulsive consumption of a substance or by certain compulsive behaviour. Both behaviour types are rewarding in the short term but may also have associated negative effects, especially in the long term.

The path to addiction is familiar to anyone who has been a smoker or who has flirted with alcohol or cannabis. The first step is normally to try the substance in question in small quantities, out of curiosity or through social influences, because it makes you feel good and/or because it helps you lose your inhibitions. Consumption is initially sporadic but, as time passes, and if it becomes a habit, it may progressively increase, both in terms of frequency and quantity. Almost without realising, you slowly start feeling a sense of need which, depending on the type of substance involved, on your lifestyle and on each individual, develops at a faster or slower pace. This is the process of becoming addicted to a given substance.

It's worth mentioning at this point that experts generally are careful with how they use the term "addiction" because, scientifically speaking, it lacks precision. Instead, they tend to use the concepts of "abuse" (referring to an excessive and compulsive consumption or practice) and "dependence" (referring to the intense feeling or sensation of the need to continue consuming or practising every so often). Though these terms put the associated relationships and pathological behaviour types in sharper focus, I shall continue to use the term "addiction" throughout this book, as this is not an academic work and all the ideas outlined above are conveniently encapsulated in this one word. Nevertheless, experts have a valid point in preferring to use the other two semantic concepts.

Though we've all got an idea of what an addiction is, its operating mechanisms (how an addiction actually works) remain, to a large extent, a mystery for science. We recognise the symptoms and effects of an addiction but are still largely unfamiliar with what actually happens, at a physiological and molecular level, in our organism to drive us to lose control and to crave something that may be highly toxic and harmful. Once again, the key to the answer is in the brain, as this is where the effects and alterations that modify our behaviour are generated. Whereas research on this subject can be traced back several decades, it is only now that strong evidence is appearing to enable certain hypotheses on this discipline to be put forward. Questions on the subject, however, still outnumber answers.

Amongst other effects, all substances considered to be addictive have the capacity to increase dopamine activity in various areas of the brain. And yes, once again we find ourselves talking about dopamine, that same neurotransmitter we spoke about before. This is logical when you consider that dopamine is the chemical that triggers a large number of nerve cells into action, including those related to sensations of pleasure and in the reward circuit.

Historically, it was believed that the repetitive consumption of addictive substances over long periods of time may have the effect of progressively numbing dopamine receptors, creating a kind of resistance to it, as is the case with insulin and leptin. It could be said that, after being incessantly bombarded by this neurotransmitter, the receptors grow accustomed to its presence and, consequently, dopamine concentration in the brain needs to be increasingly higher for pleasure levels to be maintained. In other words, if dopamine concentration is not sufficiently high in certain areas of the brain which control motivation and feelings of desire, then this is when withdrawal symptoms, dependence and compulsive consumption enter the fray. One might say that the dopaminergic neurons, those which, amongst other things, drive us to take a decision and to take action, are requesting more and more dopamine to sate their appetite.

Later research, however, revealed that this model is not only incomplete but probably inaccurate. Addiction is a far more complex phenomenon than this, with more neurotransmitters influencing the system (for example, cannabinoids). The most likely explanation is that it involves a diverse combination of biochemical and genetic mechanisms.

More recent hypotheses have developed models based on epigenetic modifications which may generate all these substances. Epigenetics, a relatively new branch of science attracting a great deal of attention and resources, may hold a lot of promise for a multitude of medical applications. An in-depth look into epigenetics would require a series of long and technical explanations, so I will merely try to summarise the concept here to give you a general idea of what's behind it.

Epigenetic factors are gene regulatory mechanisms, normally molecules which do not in themselves form part of genes but which impact on how they work. These molecules are susceptible to change triggered by environmental or external factors. Depending on the configuration and state of these molecules, genes may suffer functional alterations. Certain regulatory mechanisms (epigenetic factors) even dictate gene expression; in other words, they switch genes on and off, and I'm sure you already know that genes are the information units of the genome, which house the basic instructions for the whole of our body, including the synthesis of proteins and hormones.

In recent times, epigenetics has secured a high media profile due to the fact that numerous genes are being discovered to be associated with certain diseases, and that it may be possible in the relatively near future to control the expression of these genes using epigenetic mechanisms. The molecules of this type "surrounding" the genes would simple need to be manipulated as required. The possibilities here are immense, as this technology would enable therapies to be designed to prevent many of these diseases and even to combat them. However, for the moment, we're talking of nothing more than possibilities.

So let's get back to the present. We are, in fact, subject to environmental factors which are also capable of modifying the molecules mentioned above. If these molecules cause some of the genes involved in the synthesis of certain hormones and proteins to be activated, this may have a significant effect. In turn, if these newly synthesized hormones and proteins are capable of altering our physiology, this could give rise to cellular or neuronal changes that translate into major behavioural shifts, such as those observed during withdrawal syndrome or in the failure to control compulsive behaviour. In other words, addiction.

Some experts conducting research in this area believe the Delta-FOSB gene to be directly associated with addiction. Furthermore, they also believe to have proved that this relation goes beyond simple association and is, effectively, a cause-effect relationship. Hypotheses have been put forward suggesting that a high and repetitive consumption of hedonic foodstuffs could give rise to the previously mentioned epigenetic molecular changes, which in turn would provoke a progressive activation of Delta-FOSB genes, the activity of which could seriously affect specific areas of the brain. Such damage may even be irreversible, which would give substance to the widely-held belief that an addiction is practically impossible to cure (which does not mean it can't be treated or that we can't learn to remove it from our lives and lead a normal life, as is the case with thousands of recovered addicts).

Back to real size

In addition to enabling new therapies to be designed, the fledgling and exciting world of research into the epigenetic model and the molecular mechanisms of addiction could also help scientists to characterise and pinpoint the problem, i.e. to really understand exactly what it is and how it comes about. But for now, let's put this to one side and refocus on the clinical aspect of this issue, the one that can most readily help us to understand the phenomenon. The different theories espoused by healthcare professionals when dealing with their patients and prescribing different treatments are rooted in this aspect.

Generally speaking, addictions are treated by psychiatrists, so it is reasonable for us to approach the subject from the perspective of this same medical discipline. To do so, we'll use the *Diagnostic and Statistical Manual of Mental Disorders*, or DSM, a reference book of psychiatry published by the American Psychiatric Association (APA) and used throughout the world for diagnosis of the most important mental disorders. This hefty tome of around 1,000 pages classifies mental disorders and provides clear descriptions of the diagnostic categories for clinical experts and health science researchers to be able to diagnose, study and exchange information and treat these disorders. The DSM is now in its fifth edition (DSM-5), published in May 2013.

Most of the content of the DSM-5 in relation to addictions refers to situations resulting from consumption of the substances that most commonly come to mind as drugs, such as tobacco, alcohol, cocaine and cannabis. However, if we look through the list of contents, there is also a specific section on eating behaviour disorders which mentions certain well-known pathologies such as bulimia and anorexia, and other lesser-known ones such as pica and rumination syndrome. But "food addiction" *per se*? Not a word. The concept which comes closest to this would be binge eating, another reasonably well-known disorder which, as the term itself indicates, refers to the habit of eating much more than is necessary in an uncontrolled fashion. The DSM-5, as it does for all psychiatric disorders, lists reference behaviour patterns for binge eating to provide healthcare professionals with the information to decide whether their patient is really suffering from this disorder or not.

The 5 behaviour types associated with binge eating are:

1. Eating much faster than normal.
2. Eating until uncomfortably full.
3. Eating large quantities of food without feeling physically hungry.
4. Eating alone out of shame at the amount you are eating.
5. Feeling disgusted with yourself, with a subsequent feeling of depression or guilt.

The manual also provides other details to enable a correct diagnosis, such as frequency (at least once a week), severity and other associated behaviour types, amongst other things.

However, this psychiatric perspective of binge eating only covers a very limited area of the overall concept of what can possibly be called "food addiction". In the DSM-5, binge eating focuses exclusively on one type of compulsive behaviour, without going any further into other psychological and physiological aspects which may help characterise the phenomenon and identify possible treatments.

Leaving eating disorders momentarily to one side and returning to what the DSM has to say on addictive substances, parallels and comparisons may be drawn to potentially help us with our inquiries. This part of the manual provides the reader with a comprehensive overview of the most commonly used substances, from the most widely accepted (coffee) to the hardest (heroin), including in most cases a list of 10 or 12 behaviour types and symptoms associated with each one. This is of great use, as it can be easily understood and used to make a diagnosis.

As you've probably imagined, food is not included in this list of addictive substances. However, if we analyse the symptoms and details of some of the eating disorders which are included (for example, binge eating or bulimia nervosa), it's not difficult to draw parallels with alcohol or cocaine addiction.

Fortunately, not all overweight people suffer from eating disorders. Which raises an interesting question: can certain similarities be found among obese people who do not suffer from any of these pathologies? People who have not been diagnosed with any type of eating disorder but who wage a daily battle against excess weight? Well, the truth is that although it's an attractive and interesting idea, on deeper analysis, a series of problems arise. For example, if we're looking for a substance they may be addicted to, what would that equivalent addictive substance be? Sugar? Fat? Salt? All of them? Complex foods? And if everyone has access to these foods, why don't we all become addicted to them? Where do we draw the line between use and the abuse that leads to addiction?

Tests in animals clearly indicate that rats may especially develop an addiction to foods with a high sugar or fat content. However, this issue seems to be considerably more complex in humans. Opinion is divided on the issue, with no prevailing consensus on such a recent approach. Furthermore, not much work has been done to date on studying which are the supposedly most addictive foods, and the work that has been done on the issue has been based on the subjective evaluations of the subjects under study. As expected, results show significant variation depending on the dietary culture of each region and on each individual's eating history, but in general, the foods listed below are those which patients generally say are the most addictive:

- Chocolate, sweets, pastries, biscuits, ice-cream and desserts.

- Intensely-flavoured and rapidly-absorbed snack foods (crisps, corn and potato snacks, crackers, etc.).

- Fast food (pizza, pre-cooked and battered foods, etc.)

- Pasta, bread and rice.

One way of looking further into these concepts and ideas may be to identify the different aspects and symptoms normally taken into account in commonly and well-known addictive substances and to compare them with what happens in the case of foods, drawing and identifying subsequent parallels and similarities. For example, one interesting way of doing this is to use magnetic resonance imaging (fMRI) to observe neural response to images or representations of this type of highly appetising and palatable food, and to compare it to neural response to images of addictive substances (alcohol, tobacco, cocaine, etc.). Research of this type has shown that in both cases, many areas of the brain related to reward are activated, with the dopaminergic system leading the way. Findings have also revealed that some areas are activated in one case but not in the other, and vice-versa. Thus, although certain findings do overlap or coincide, there are also differences, both in terms of the intensity of neural activity and in the areas where this activity is seen to take place. In any case, to date, few studies have been conducted on this subject, and those that have are rather heterogeneous.

Another more qualitative method of comparison with a more clinical approach is to use the criteria that the DSM-5 proposes to assess addiction to substances and drugs. Below are the 11 symptoms of reference for addiction to a given substance:

1. Consumption in large amounts or over a long period.

2. Persistent desire or unsuccessful efforts to cut down consumption.

3. A great deal of time spent on activities necessary for consumption or on consumption itself.

4. Craving or a strong desire or urge to consume.

5. Recurrent consumption resulting in a failure to fulfil major role obligations.

6. Continued consumption despite persistent and recurrent personal or interpersonal problems.

7. Important activities are given up or reduced because of consumption.

8. Consumption in physically hazardous situations.

9. Continued consumption despite knowledge of having persistent or recurrent physical or psychological problems.

10. Tolerance (need to increase consumption over time).

11. Withdrawal syndrome.

According to the DSM, if two or more of these symptoms are present for at least one year and accompanied by repeated and significant distress or impaired functioning, then the situation could be regarded as the beginning of an addiction to a particular substance.

And using this type of comparison, what do we find? A mixed bag. As mentioned above, several of these symptoms are found amongst people suffering from an eating disorder such as binge eating or anorexia, but findings are more heterogeneous amongst obese people who do not suffer from any such disorder. Furthermore, the results depend to a large extent on which of the 11 symptoms we are talking about. For example, there is considerable evidence that the following four symptoms are frequently to be found amongst a large number of people who often overeat:

1. Consumption in large amounts or over a long period.

2. Persistent desire or unsuccessful efforts to cut down consumption.

4. Craving or a strong desire or urge to consume.

9. Continued consumption despite knowledge of having persistent or recurrent physical or psychological problems.

Conversely, there is no solid proof with regard to the other seven symptoms, either because the findings obtained have been inconclusive or because specific studies on the issue have yet to be conducted.

From an objective perspective, and in accordance with the DSM-5 manual itself, the presence of 2 or 3 of these symptoms (in addition to the previously mentioned marked sense of distress) would indicate a minor disorder, 4 or 5 of the symptoms would indicate a moderate disorder and 6 or more symptoms, a severe disorder. However, things are not as straightforward as that. To get an idea of the kind of doubts which arise in scientists' minds when using this type of comparison, the last symptom (withdrawal syndrome) provides a good illustration of the difficulties science is up against. Remember... we're talking here about hunger or appetite, so the question arises of where hunger induced by the need for energy or nutrition ends, and where hedonic hunger, or hunger for reasons related to a supposed addiction, begins.

Due to these difficulties, some experts are not particularly willing to accept these hypotheses. They believe that the assessment of the different symptoms is not sufficiently well structured and may be open to subjectivity, particularly in the case of self-assessment, i.e. when the patient is left to make an assessment of his or her own case. Others believe that some of the symptoms are not applicable, as there is no scientific proof of their existence when talking about food. This is especially so in the case of certain key symptoms (such as withdrawal syndrome or tolerance) related to the biochemical processes and mechanisms behind addiction. In their opinion, more evidence is required to confirm their existence.

The most ardent critics of this type of comparison also point out that another factor common to addictive substances but missing in this case is the risk of acute intoxication. Especially high consumption of certain substances may have serious or even fatal consequences for an individual's health, as consumers of heroin and cocaine know only too well, but it is equally true that this is not the case in other substances such as tobacco.

It is, therefore, fair to say that although this type of comparison reveals several overlapping areas, coincidences and aspects in common, there are also some important differences. Consequently, for the moment, no clear consensus on the issue can be said to exist. It seems that many experts have yet to form an opinion on this issue, so the controversy continues. On the basis of the considerable bibliography and findings from initial scientific studies on the subject, the situation can be summarised as follows: while some people believe that we are talking of two different phenomena because not all the required conditions are strictly met, others think that things are not that black and white and, as medicine is not a mathematical science, that the idea of applying the concepts and approaches related to addiction may prove useful in the battle against obesity.

Just out of curiosity, you may be interested to know that certain parallels can also be drawn between the potentiality of food addiction and other types of disorders cited in the DSM-5 but not related to addictive substances, e.g. pathological gambling, kleptomania, pyromania and other such lesser-known disorders. Practically all of them present symptoms familiar to some overweight people, such as unsuccessful attempts to control the habit and the concern and distress felt by the person affected.

In any case, irrespective of these apparent similarities with other pathologies, the fact is that psychiatry has yet to formally acknowledge the concept of "food addiction disorder" or something similar. Or rather, this concept has yet to find its way into the bibliographical references most widely used by psychiatrists, as other well-known and treated eating disorders have existed there for some time. Regardless, a series of interesting initiatives are currently being taken forward – for the moment, albeit isolated ones at a nascent stage and in need of further development and refinement – to be able to diagnose and treat pathologies of this nature.

One of the most interesting initiatives, and probably the one that has most contributed to disseminating the theory of food addiction, was developed by researchers at the University of Yale. In 2009, they drew up a specific questionnaire on food addiction, based on the DSM-IV lists of symptoms associated with substance dependence. This initially singular and unusual proposal aroused increasing interest in scientists, to the point where it has become a respected source of reference. Nowadays, the so-called *Yale Food Addiction Scale* (YFAS) is a well-known and widely used tool, and is cited in practically all research work on the subject.

The original questionnaire consisted of 25 items intended to be the equivalent of those related to substance abuse. A modified version was later drawn up with nine items designed to make the questionnaire easier to use in large-scale epidemiological studies. These items are listed below:

1. I find myself consuming certain foods even though I am no longer hungry.
2. I worry about cutting down on certain foods.
3. I feel sluggish or fatigued from overeating.
4. I have spent time dealing with negative feelings from overeating certain foods, instead of spending time in important activities such as time with family, friends, work or recreation.
5. I have had physical withdrawal symptoms such as agitation and anxiety when I cut down on certain foods (do NOT include caffeinated drinks: coffee, tea, cola, energy drinks, etc.).
6. I kept consuming the same types or amounts of food despite significant physical and/or emotional problems related to my eating.
7. Eating the same amount of food does not reduce negative emotions or increase pleasurable feelings the way it used to.

8. My behaviour with respect to food and eating causes me significant distress.
9. Issues related to food and eating decrease my ability to function effectively (daily routine, job/school, social or family activities, health difficulties).

This version is not only the most widely used but also the one which has had the greatest impact among the health community. A children's version of the questionnaire also exists.

Can you identify with one or more of these symptoms? You should know that, broadly speaking, the diagnosis is considered as positive if two conditions have been maintained over the last 12 months: firstly, that at least one of the last two symptoms (items 8 & 9) has been identified at least twice a week, and secondly, that at least 3 of the 7 remaining symptoms (items 1 to 7) have been identified with similar frequency. As in the case of addictive substances, the higher the number of symptoms present, the more severe the disorder is considered to be.

The first studies conducted using this methodology show that the possible prevalence of the hypothetical pathology of food addiction may be considered as significant, especially among adult obese people (it is estimated that up to one fifth of the obese population may suffer from this possible pathology). Surprisingly, findings also reveal that one in ten normal weight people may also suffer from it. Findings from these first studies in relation to overweight children and teenagers are of even more concern, revealing that anything between one third and two thirds of this collective may be affected.

Once again, no clear consensus on the validity of this claim can be said to exist. Far from it, in fact. Advocates of the YFAS claim these incidence rates to be clear evidence of the existence of foods capable of creating addiction and which could be at the root of the global epidemic of obesity. Conversely, its detractors claim that too many overweight people fail to comply with its findings, thereby making it difficult to consider the YFAS as clinically useful and effective.

In short, only time and science will tell if addiction to food (or something similar) will feature amongst the pages of future editions of the DSM, with a list of symptoms resembling that of the YFAS. If so, this would give significant momentum to the psychiatric perspective of the treatment of obesity, a potentially new and powerful front line to increase the possibilities of victory in this seemingly endless battle.

Stress and eating

At this point, then, the initial model outlined in previous chapters of this book, where the intake of food has been analysed from a homeostatic (eating to cover energy needs) and a hedonic (eating for pleasure) perspective, starts to become a little blurred. Though this model may be useful to clarify how our brain works in terms of managing appetite, in reality, the different parts of the brain do not function independently from each other. Just the opposite, in fact. There is a constant and complex pattern of interrelation among them, despite the fact that each individual part may specialise in certain specific tasks.

There are, without doubt, certain foods that provide us with a unique and particular sense of pleasure when we eat them. Likewise, it may be possible to prove that those foods are addictive. However, it must be remembered that eating, both now and in the past, has always played a fundamental role in human society. Eating is an important social act, an occasion used not only to acquire energy and nutrients but to be with family, friends and workmates. Furthermore, as we shall see in more detail in the next section, the subtleties and nuances used in food advertising are of the highest order. Food marketing has created a world in which the food we buy and store at home is no longer a mere source of energy but an integral element of social status.

In short, eating has become a very neurologically complex process. Emotions and physiological needs, brain and metabolism, neurons and the digestive system... all these dual factors are subtly but clearly interwoven. It is, therefore, not unreasonable to deduce that the different variables affecting this world of emotions and feelings, including our social relations and how we perceive the world around us, may influence our decision-making process with regard to eating. They may even be the driving force behind our eating habits, the prime movers of those semi-pathological and undesirable situations that healthcare professionals come up against on an ever more frequent basis.

If asked to think of an intense and everyday emotion affecting a lot of people in the world, then stress would likely be one of the first to come to mind. Stress is one of the ailments most frequently diagnosed by doctors and probably one of the trademark characteristics of modern life in the developed world. To one extent or another, practically all of us have suffered from stress at some time in our life: that feeling of deep concern and anguish caused by rushing, by a lack of time, by unsolved problems and/or by constant anxiety. However, stress is nothing new; it's been with us since ancient times and is really nothing more than a reaction of the body to prepare for a situation it perceives as threatening or which is going to require a special or extraordinary effort. When confronted by this type of alert or emergency situation, this natural bodily reaction has ensured the survival over time of a large number of living beings.

From the somatic perspective, stress is a chain reaction, set in motion from the central nervous system, which triggers significant physiological, psychological and behavioural changes over a limited period of time. A series of molecules and elements are secreted to activate biochemical processes which bring about important changes in nervous and neural activity, manifest in us as nervousness, apprehension, an increase in heartbeat, pupil dilation, sweating, goose pimples, increased blood pressure and reduced libido, amongst other features. It's important to understand that all these changes occur with one sole objective; to ensure the required physiological resources reach the places in the body where they are most needed, diverting, where necessary, the flow of blood to the heart, muscles and brain.

For example, imagine you hear a sound that makes you suspect the presence of a dangerous predator. Your body becomes focused, your heartbeat starts to race, your muscles tense up and everything gets ready to take immediate action (to run away or to defend yourself) and to recover as soon as possible from a potential damage-inflicting confrontation. Logically, this state will continue for as long as the situation remains the same, or whilst there is a high possibility that the body will have to respond to an experience which places high demands on it. Finally, once the mystery has been revealed – hopefully, it was nothing more than a rodent scurrying amongst the bushes – all this biochemical activity stops and may even be reversed, causing the body and the metabolism to go back to normal.

So, the process of stress, as described above, is not in itself the problem, as it is an important and necessary physiological reaction. The problem comes when the length and frequency of this process increases to extremes that can be described as abnormal. As is the case with inflammation – a normal and necessary reaction to repair specific damage in the body, but a pathological reaction if it's continuously present – the difficulties arise when stress is no longer something occasional but a chronic condition. It is then when our body begins to have to tolerate the negative side of stress.

This latter type of stress is a characteristic feature of our modern lifestyle. Nowadays, few of us are openly exposed to extremely dangerous or emergency situations for which the body must prepare itself and respond to rapidly. Just the opposite, in fact: modern society is safer than ever, and we are exposed to very few real risks. We live, however, in a permanent state of stress. Thoughts and concerns run constantly through our minds without us ever finding any real solutions to them. Everything gets tied up together and magnified, drowning us in a sea of anxiety with no clear beginning or end and extremely difficult to control. This universe we create in our head is the consequence of the complexity of today's lifestyle; one which, although perhaps no more difficult than yesteryear's, is certainly much more nuanced. A social model riddled with nagging uncertainties which have no black-and-white or yes-and-no solutions, a universe in which human relations have reached a previously unknown level of sophistication.

In all this, findings of epidemiological studies frequently reveal that chronic stress levels amongst obese people are higher than average. This may seem paradoxical, as stress usually blocks off or slows down basic physiological needs such as eating (and hunger-related signals) to be able to focus on what is really important and urgent, i.e. taking the required action. In fact, the feeling of having a knot in your stomach and not feeling hungry in tense situations is something we're all familiar with. So, what's the explanation for this? Why aren't people who are continually stressed thinner?

The answer can be found in the previous chapters of this book dealing with the reasons why we eat, and, of course, in clinical trials conducted on the subject. Studies have shown that animals also experience that knot-in-the-stomach feeling, as the stress provoked in them by experimenters alters their food intake and usually leads to them eating less than normal of the food provided for them (a specific feed given to them every day). However, when the components of that same feed are modified in such a way as to raise its reward factor (in other words, when the feed becomes highly palatable and flavourful, particularly by adding sugar), the animals' response to stress is exactly the opposite: their consumption increases.

The reasons behind this apparent contradiction can be found both in the biochemical mechanisms and the psychological processes involved. One of the areas of the brain involved in responding to stress is found in the hypothalamus. If you remember from previous chapters of this book, the hypothalamus is also the area of the brain that regulates our energy homeostasis to ensure we don't run out of "fuel", with neural activity triggering appetite or satiety and compelling us to eat or to stop eating. Amongst many other processes, stress generates an enormous amount of biochemical compounds and hormones, one of which, cortisol, deserves special mention. Cortisol, also known as "the stress hormone", belongs to the family of glucocorticoids, and is closely connected to our circadian rhythms. The highest concentration levels of cortisol are therefore to be found when we get up, and the lowest, when we go to bed.

How is this hormone related to appetite and the desire to eat? Well, for cortisol (and other glucocorticoids) to be secreted, another hormone must first be secreted to trigger a type of chain reaction, the end result of which is the release of glucocorticoids and cortisol. We now know that one of the places where this trigger hormone is produced is the hypothalamus. Bearing this in mind, let's explain the situation using an analogy: when the hypothalamus is busy producing this trigger hormone, the neurons responsible for arousing our homeostatic appetite would seem to be reluctant to make us feel hungry and remind us that we need to eat.

On the other hand, what happens in other parts of the brain, those associated with the reward circuit in relation to highly palatable foods, is another story. It would seem that us humans are no different to rats in that our consumption of palatable food goes up when we are subjected to situations of stress, and our response to a high cortisol concentration is coherent with this (and contrary to the perspective of homeostatic eating). Experts have found that cortisol concentration levels are higher in people who suffer from eating disorders such as binge eating and bulimia. Furthermore, several studies have also associated a high reactivity to cortisol (large-scale secretion in response to stress) with a greater tendency to consume high reward foods. Thus, it is clear that in the case of high reward foods, the stress-induced knot-in-the-stomach factor does not come into play. Just the opposite, in fact: to a certain extent, it would seem that we search out that little moment of pleasure those foods provide us with to compensate for the stress we are under.

To make matters worse, some studies associate the large-scale presence of this hormone over long periods of time with various metabolic imbalances, especially when it acts in synergy with high insulin concentrations (hyperinsulinemia). In these cases, creation of body fat is often seen to increase, together with a difficulty to use that fat as an energy source. In other words, it can also be said that people suffering from stress are less effective at burning calories than people who aren't suffering from stress.

The responses to this undesirable and problematic situation are once again to be found in the network of biochemical processes within our organism. Cortisol appears to interact with other hormones such as insulin and leptin and, in doing so, hinders the possible interactions of those two hormones with other compounds related to their normal functions. When cortisol is continuously and repeatedly present, it may imbalance the whole system. What's more, researchers have found that cortisol may be associated with resistance to both of these hormones (though this is not known for certain), and therefore with the consequences that arise from this, as seen in previous chapters of this book.

And to cap it all, excess cortisol levels lead to increased concentration of neuropeptide Y (NPY) and ghrelin, and also inhibit the release of insulin, impeding the emission of satiety signals in the corresponding neurons which would help us combat the desire to eat.

The fact that stress can be considered another of those factors which create a vicious circle and contribute to the obesity loop is an additional handicap. Science has known for some time that compensatory addictive substances such as drugs and alcohol are more likely to be used when people confront elements and situations considered to be negative. Chronic stress, with its associated anguish and interminable distress, can be considered a negative situation. Thus, if food addiction and drug addiction really do have aspects in common, then the connections would be evident. Moreover, overweight people frequently go on strict diets, or set themselves stringent food and calorie restrictions, which often make them feel they're perpetually missing out on something and which may, as a side-effect, generate in them a feeling of tension and anguish throughout most of the day.

Analysis of brain activity suggests that when these two factors (restriction + stress) are present at the same time, reward derived from hedonic eating diminishes. In other words, a larger quantity of hedonic foods is required to sate a person's expectations. At the same time, receptivity to opioids, another type of neurotransmitter related to addiction, increases. Like dopamine, opioids are endowed with the capacity to drive us to look for a particular substance and to make us want to consume it to further activate the reward circuit.

So, as you can see, the victors once again are those neurotransmitters which activate the neurons which make us decide to repeatedly and uncontrollably consume. And all this despite the fact that the decision taken may not be the one most to our liking. If this behaviour repeats itself time and again over a period of years, it may even turn into a serious disorder.

For obvious reasons, it is difficult to discuss the subject of stress without eventually mentioning psychological disorders of a similar, though more serious, condition such as depression. You really don't need to be a specialist to imagine that in the case of depression, the problem becomes more acute and considerably more complicated. The incidence of depression among obese people is particularly high, and recent research has revealed the impact of the increase in cortisol and inflammation markers in unbalancing the neuroendocrinological system.

Future studies are likely to associate more psychiatric and psychological pathologies with obesity. In view of the ever clearer link between obesity and the brain, and with further evidence that obesity is firmly rooted in our universe of feelings and emotions, the pathways between them can be expected to intersect much more than what we had imagined to date.

REFERENCES

'It's on your conscience all the time': a systematic review of qualitative studies examining views on obesity among young people aged 12-18 years in the UK (Rees et al, 2014)

Just as smart but not as successful: obese students obtain lower school grades but equivalent test scores to nonobese students (MacCann et al, 2013)

Are overweight and obese youths more often bullied by their peers? A meta-analysis on the correlation between weight status and bullying (2015)

The affective and interpersonal consequences of obesity (Levine et al, 2015)

Perceived Weight Discrimination and Changes in Weight, Waist circumference, and Weight Status (Jackson et al, 2014)

The stigma of obesity in the general public and its implications for public health - a systematic review (Sikorski et al, 2011)

Residual stigma: psychological distress among the formerly overweight (Levy et al, 2012)

Who is to blame for the rise in obesity? (Lusk et al, 2013)

Primum non nocere: obesity stigma and public health (Vartanian et al, 2013)

Beliefs, attitudes and phobias among medical and psychology students towards people with obesity (Soto et al, 2014)

Weight bias among UK trainee dietitians, doctors, nurses and nutritionists (Swift et al, 2013)

The academic penalty for gaining weight: a longitudinal, change-in-change analysis of BMI and perceived academic ability in middle school students (Kenney et al, 2015)

Weight bias in 2001 versus 2013: Contradictory attitudes among obesity researchers and health professionals (Tomiyama et al, 2014)

Impact of Physician BMI on Obesity Care and Beliefs (Bleich et al, 2012)

The effect of physicians' body weight on patient attitudes: implications for physician selection, trust and adherence to medical advice (Puhl et al, 2013)

Physicians build less rapport with obese patients (Gudzune et al, 2013)

Public reactions to obesity-related health campaigns: a randomized controlled trial (Puhl et al, 2013)

Fighting obesity or obese persons? Public perceptions of obesity-related health messages (Puhl et al, 2013)

Effects of messages from a media campaign to increase public awareness of childhood obesity (Barry et al, 2014)

Low Message Sensation Health Promotion Videos Are Better Remembered and Activate Areas of the Brain Associated with Memory Encoding (Seelig et al, 2014)

Fatness predicts decreased physical activity and increased sedentary time, but not vice versa: support from a longitudinal study in 8- to 11-year-old children (Hjorth et al, 2013)

Fatness leads to inactivity, but inactivity does not lead to fatness: a longitudinal study in children (Metcalf, 2010)

Eating on impulse: the relation between overweight and food-specific inhibitory control (Houben et al, 2014)

Food quality and motivation: a refined low-fat diet induces obesity and impairs performance on a progressive ratio schedule of instrumental lever pressing in rats (Blaisdell y otros 2014)

Natural Rewards, Neuroplasticity, and Non-Drug Addictions (CM Olsen, 2011)

The Neurobiology of Addiction: Where We Have Been and Where We Are Going (Koob, 2009)

Epigenetic mechanisms of drug addiction (Nestler, 2013)

Evidence for sugar addiction: Behavioral and neurochemical effects of intermittent, excessive sugar intake (Avena, 2008)

Food Cravings in a College Population (Weingarten et al, 1991)

Food cravings, food intake, and weight status in a community-based sample population (Chao et al, 2014)

Rice and sushi cravings: A preliminary study of food craving among Japanese females (Komatsu , 2008)

Food liking and craving: A cross-cultural approach (Zellner et al, 1999)

Food cravings and energy regulation: the characteristics of craved foods and their relationship with eating behaviors and weight change during 6 months of dietary energy restriction (Gilhooly et al, 2007)

Which foods may be addictive? The roles of processing, fat content, and glycemic load (Schulte et al, 2015)

Excessive Sugar Consumption May Be a Difficult Habit to Break: A View From the Brain and Body (Tryon y otros)

The contribution of brain reward circuits to the obesity epidemic (Stice et al, 2012)

The generation and inhibition of hedonically-driven food intake: Behavioral and neurophysiological determinants in healthy weight individuals (Ely et al, 2013)

Food Addiction in the Light of DSM-5 (Meule, 2014)

Food and drug cues activate similar brain regions: a meta-analysis of functional MRI studies (Tang et al, 2012)

Reward processing in obesity, substance addiction and non-substance addiction (García et al, 2015)

A Qualitative Study of Binge Eating and Obesity From an Addiction Perspective (Curtis et al, 2014)

Obesity and the brain: how convincing is the addiction model? (Ziauddeen et al, 2012)

Is food addiction a valid and useful concept? (Ziauddeen et al,2013)

Eating addiction", rather than "food addiction", better captures addictive-like eating behavior (Hebebrand et al, 2014)

The Neurobiological Underpinnings of Obesity and Binge Eating: A Rationale for Adopting the Food Addiction Model (Smith et al, 2012)

Five years of the Yale Food Addiction Scale: Taking stock and moving forward (Meule, 2014)

The Prevalence of Food Addiction as Assessed by the Yale Food Addiction Scale: A Systematic Review (Pursey et al, 2014)

Food-addiction scale measurement in 2 cohorts of middle-aged and older women (2014)

Food Addiction in Overweight and Obese Adolescents Seeking Weight-loss Treatment (2015)

A new insight into food addiction in childhood obesity (2014)

Rationale and Consequences of Reclassifying Obesity as an Addictive Disorder: Neurobiology, Food Environment and Social Policy Perspectives (Allen et al, 2012)

The Addiction Potential of Hyperpalatable Foods (Gearhart et al, 2011)

Striatocortical pathway dysfunction in addiction and obesity: differences and similarities (Tomasi et al, 2013)

Obesity Is Associated with Decreased μ-Opioid But Unaltered Dopamine D2 Receptor Availability in the Brain (Karlsson et al, 2015)

The association of "food addiction" with disordered eating and body mass index (Geardhart et al, 2014)

How prevalent is "food addiction"? (Meule, 2011)

Obesity and the brain: how convincing is the addiction model? (Ziaudeen et al, 2012)

Clearing the Confusion around Processed Food Addiction (Ifland et al, 2015)

Stress as a common risk factor for obesity and addiction (Sinha et al, 2013)

Stress augments food 'wanting' and energy intake in visceral overweight subjects in the absence of hunger (Lemmens et al, 2011)

Stress, eating and the reward system (Adam et al, 2007)

Chronic stress exposure may affect the brain's response to high calorie food cues and predispose to obesogenic eating habits (Tryon et al, 2013)

Daily Stressors, Past Depression, and Metabolic Responses to High-Fat Meals: A Novel Path to Obesity (Kiecolt-Glaser et al, 2014)

Eating behavior and stress: a pathway to obesity (Sominsky et al, 2014)

Acute stress and food-related reward activation in the brain during food choice during eating in the absence of hunger (Born et al, 2010)

Immediate effects of chocolate on experimentally induced mood states (Macht, 2007)

Metabolic disturbances connecting obesity and depression (Fulton et al, 2013)

Depression and inflammation: Examining the link (Almond, 2013)

2.3. A DUPED BRAIN

Unlike plants, an animal's metabolism is not capable of obtaining energy from sunlight, inorganic elements or other such sources. To obtain energy, we need to absorb organic elements, generally using other living beings as a supply source, as our existence depends on sourcing energy. It could therefore be argued that obtaining diverse organic matter from other living beings is absolutely essential for our survival, which would explain why most animals are so well prepared to seek out and obtain food and the considerable resources we dedicate to it.

The main (though not the only) drivers behind the evolution of most species have fundamentally been their effectiveness in seeking out food and in not falling prey to others. Focusing on the first of these factors and, more particularly, on mammals, the category of animal closest to man in evolutionary terms, most of them spend just about all their time doing precisely this. Gorillas have been estimated to spend around ten hours per day eating, whilst elephants need to spend just about all their time searching for food and eating to secure the 100+ kilograms of vegetable matter their organism requires.

In its quest for a deeper insight into the correlation between how much food animals need and the resources they need to obtain it, one of the concerns of the scientific community has been to analyse different variables related to this issue using mathematical and numerical models. By studying the relation between the size of a mammal, the size of its brain, the type of food it requires and the time spent seeking out and obtaining that food, scientists have been able to explain and anticipate this correlation with reasonable accuracy. As a result, we can now say with some certainty that what our predecessors ate influenced the evolutionary history of the exceptional level of human intelligence.

I shall attempt to illustrate the relationship between all these variables by providing more detailed explanations, more examples and offering up some ideas.

As you will no doubt remember from the first part of this book, the amount of energy consumed by neurons is exceptionally high compared to that consumed by other cell types. Not only the neurons in the human brain but those of any animal. It follows then that although the energy obtained from food is carefully distributed throughout the body, it is channelled through to the brain, a primary organ, on a priority basis. Logically, the energy requirements of the brain depend on the number of neurons it houses: the greater the number of neurons, the more energy is required. On the other hand, the greater the number of neurons it houses, the more complex the brain becomes and the greater its capacity to develop a higher degree of intelligence, or at least, a greater cognitive and neural complexity. All this may contribute to a greater degree of effectiveness in looking for food.

At the same time, the requirements of the other parts of the body are obviously not neglected by the metabolism, and energy is delivered to our organs, muscles, tissue and bones. In this respect, the bigger the animal, the greater the joint energy requirements of all these body parts. Size may also be a useful factor in capturing prey more effectively (quicker, stronger, etc.).

Another consideration is that although foods of animal origin generally provide more energy and nutrients that those of vegetable origin, they are also more difficult to obtain and invariably require more neuronal energy (though not always, as good muscles and teeth are sometimes more than enough). Likewise, though vegetable matter may be easier to obtain (at least in favourable climates), more of it is normally required to deliver the same energy values. Furthermore, driven by their tremendous need for food, herbivores need to be almost constantly on the move after decimating the resources of the area where they have been, as is the case in the annual migration of elephants and other such animals.

As you can no doubt appreciate, all these factors together weave a rather complex pattern of relations, and over many thousands of years, evolution has seen to it that these factors are balanced out in each ecosystem and for each species, including the time spent looking for and eating food. Taking all this into consideration and converting it into equations and mathematical models, experts can calculate the time required for different species to seek out and eat the food they need on the basis of their body and brain size.

For example, it has been estimated that a 120 kg primate needs to spend at least 8 hours per day looking for and eating food to provide its neurons with enough energy. More or less the equivalent in hours of a complete working day. These calculations and models are quite accurate when applied to baboons, orangutans and gorillas in their natural habitat but not, as you are no doubt thinking, to human beings.

Our brain is a masterful tool, providing us with the intelligence and the ingenuity not only to look for and find food but many other things as well. At the same time, as so many neurons are housed there, it also needs a lot of energy. When human beings depended exclusively on the resources present in our environment to feed all those neurons, we only had two options: either to dedicate much more than eight hours a day to looking for and securing food (which wouldn't leave time for anything else, as is the case with some herbivores), or to resort to other more energy-dense foods. This is precisely why many experts believe that access to meat and the mastery of fire, which made it possible for man to cook meat and facilitate its digestion, have played a key role in enabling us to become what we have become and to have developed the brain we now have.

In any case, all these studies have shown that, even in the case of finding more energy-dense foods, time spent on feeding is of great importance in all species, including ours. It's likely that our nearest ancestors didn't spend as long as gorillas or elephants but undoubtedly spent many hours looking for nutritious foods, probably gathering, fishing and hunting. It's also reasonably certain that this was the case for many centuries, even in the most recent evolutionary periods, and that this was one of the driving forces behind us heightening and developing our intelligence and ingenuity. We can say, without any real fear of error, that a considerable number of the intellectual tasks that occupied our ancestors' brain were, apart from the most automatic functions, focused on improving the effectiveness and the efficiency of the methods and processes they used to obtain food. Likewise, there can be no doubt that food and everything related to it were uppermost in their thoughts and concerns for many thousands of years: for them, it was a simple matter of sourcing energy and nutrition or not. Of eating or starving. Of life and death.

Since then, things have moved on, and the development of technology, together with social and cultural changes, have transformed this situation completely. It could be said that this major transformation began some 10,000 years ago, when farming and livestock gradually became the main ways of obtaining food resources. The techniques used enabled energy to reach many more people, and paved the way for the availability of many more basic foodstuffs and a much simpler way of securing them. Furthermore, this lifestyle made animal and plant products available throughout most of the year, cutting out the need to travel long distances and the danger involved, for example, in hunting, not to mention the uncertainties associated, for example, with gathering.

Though agricultural life is hard and involves a lot of work and dedication, it increases the availability of food resources considerably compared to the hunting and gathering philosophy. Vegetables, fruit, pulses, cereals, milk and milk-products and meat all became available to a much higher percentage of the population. Though still largely suffering from malnutrition and shortcomings of various kinds, people now had relatively easy access to these products if they could find the infrastructure and the land required. Mind you, this still involved considerable effort and work, as the advanced production techniques of today obviously did not exist then and climate factors could quickly ruin the hard work put in over months.

However, it didn't take long for our species once again to change the rules of nature. Only this time, the change was more radical: the birth and deployment of intensive farming and livestock breeding and free trade. Production techniques became more efficient, economies of scale appeared on the scene and food manufacturers specialised, giving rise to a greater degree of mechanisation and introducing more technology. Consequently, productivity and foods derived from everyday raw materials were developed exponentially, enabling food to be distributed and marketed worldwide.

When others take responsibility for feeding us

All these changes have been particularly marked in recent decades. This transformation, together with other consequences, has made basic foodstuffs readily available for most of the population of the western world, enabling people to dedicate less of their time to ensuring their food supply. Increasing wealth and purchasing power for the citizens of any given country normally goes hand-in-hand with a reduction in the amount of resources they spend on acquiring food products. For example, in countries such as Kenya and Pakistan, almost half a typical family's income is necessarily spent purchasing food, whilst in most European countries, this figure is reduced to around one tenth of total salary, thereby enabling people to spend the rest of their income on other activities and products given increasing importance in this society, e.g. technology, leisure, social relations, etc.

In short, in the most developed societies, finding food has very much become a minor pastime. No need to hunt, gather or sow seeds... others do it for us, and a trip to the supermarket is enough for most of us. We are so used to this that it's difficult nowadays to contemplate that this, historically, is an exceptional situation. Just imagine for a second what a person from the 19th century (or even better, somebody from 2,000 years ago) would think if we transported him/her through time into a 21st century supermarket! I have absolutely no doubt that they would be left speechless, astonished by the enormous quantity and variety of products at their fingertips. In the best possible of cases, they would probably only ever have seen a dozen or so of these products together.

This revolution has not only been instrumental in how we obtain food but also in the ever-decreasing amount of time we spend preparing it. As humans, we are the only animals that subject our food to various processes of advanced transformation. Chopped, ground, mixed up, boiled, roasted... all this nowadays has been shaped and styled to the point where a whole new elaborate and complex branch of knowledge, or even an art form, has been created around such activities: cooking. In this case, however, the paradox is that at the same time as this art form has become increasingly sophisticated, there has been a drastic reduction in the amount of time the general public actually spends cooking. Another factor which has impacted heavily on this process has been the relatively recent incorporation of women into further education and the labour market. For generations, food management, for diverse cultural reasons, had been the responsibility of women. Nowadays, the fact that women are no longer available for this task has created a new need: pre-prepared food. And needless to say, the all-powerful food industry has reacted to this with characteristic speed and agility.

At this point, it's important to understand that in a free market-based economy, companies give priority to their economic indicators. In other words, and regardless of the sector, the primary objective is to make a profit, though the means and the policy used to deliver this objective may vary wildly. This business model, like all others, has its pros and cons. The advantages of the model include an obsessive concern with optimising resources, economies of scale and internationalisation, thereby making foodstuffs available and affordable for most people, dramatically reducing malnutrition levels and providing cheap energy practically worldwide. However, as the years have passed and food shortages have, relatively speaking, been overcome, we are discovering that there are also other less positive aspects attached to this model which are having a major impact on our eating habits.

The food industry is mostly controlled by ten or so enormous companies. The fact that they are so big enables them to control the whole process of product creation and distribution throughout the world, and this, in turn, gives rise to certain other issues characteristic of big companies in such large markets. The way these industrial giants maximise profits and performance for their shareholders is not by simply obtaining and distributing a wide variety of fresh foods. Costs are kept to a minimum by producing huge quantities of a very limited number of products, thereby enabling them to reduce the unit price. In other words, they take economies of scale to the extreme.

This policy may seem to be at odds with the fact that what consumers are asking for nowadays is ever greater variety. Not so. What appear to be two contradictory perspectives combine to perfection in the business model they form the basis of, a model in which the baseline is a relatively limited variety of raw materials and the final objective is an enormous diversity of end products. Or, at least, what is perceived as diversity by the consumer, as this supposed variety is, as we shall see a little later, nothing more than a figment of our imagination.

In any case, the net result of this philosophy is that, according to reliable calculations, the shelves of North American supermarkets are now stocked with over half a million different food products. One of the main components of a high percentage of these products is some kind of refined cereal grown using large-scale intensive farming methods. Additionally, these same products very often have a high added sugar content.

Another little-known but key aspect of this issue is that this model entitles companies to extra funding in the form of government subsidies, thereby monopolizing financial assistance worth millions. When government policy is drawn up to support certain economic activities considered, for one reason or another, to be priority or deserving protection, the areas which most benefit from those policies are usually those related to the primary sector, such as fishing, farming and livestock. It's true that it is sometimes necessary to protect these sectors for economic, social or environmental reasons, but it's equally true that the large food companies often take the lion's share of the money to fund their raw material production activities. This can be seen most clearly in the United States, where thousands of millions of dollars are available every year in subsidies for the production of corn.

This being the playing field, another factor of enormous importance is lobbying and the generation of opinion. The global titans of the food industry hire the best available experts – in exchange for succulent salaries – and strategically position them in carefully selected posts and activities. In this way, through representation in pressure groups and their own experts, advisors and researchers, these companies ensure their presence in congresses, campaigns, projects, social actions and any other such initiative related to food and eating. Consequently, you will almost certainly find a representative of these companies in every event or initiative of this type. This occasionally (though not as often as one would like) leads prominent members of societal organisations to denounce this type of intrusiveness which, though legal, greatly hinders their efforts to effectively focus attention on the real needs of the population without having to fight against the spurious interests and influences of these companies. In this sense, the World Health Organisation has denounced these practices on several occasions.

All this carefully organised lobbying is combined with another factor considered by these multinational giants to be equally (or more) important as their production processes: their marketing and sales processes. Few sectors spend as much money on publicity and communication as the food sector, and food companies and their products figure among the best customers of the most prestigious and expensive marketing experts in the world. To give you an idea of what we're talking about, the cereals sector usually spends twice as much on marketing as it does on raw material costs. In fact, as we saw before in the section of this book covering the reward and pleasure provided by foodstuffs designed by the food industry, each new product is developed with an in-depth market and viability study, identifying the best way to present, sell and market it throughout the world. All with the end purpose of reaching the target audience carefully defined more or less since the product was first created.

When marketing rules the brain

So, what's the brain's got to do with all of this? As explained above, for thousands of years, our brain has been designed, amongst other things, to seek out and find food to ensure our survival. Using this as a baseline, marketing experts have gone to great lengths to identify the most effective techniques and strategies for selling us those foods. This research has been conducted as thoroughly (or perhaps even more thoroughly) in the food sector as in other sectors, though the unique nature of food confers certain special features on the issue as we are about to see.

The most automatic part of our brain, or the part which works on instinct more than anything else, is triggered into action by messages from two different sources: firstly, messages in relation to the senses awoken, principally in and around our mouth and nose, by the end result of the foodstuff in question (texture, taste, smell, etc.), and secondly, messages relaying what our eyes are taking in; in other words, the appearance of the foodstuff itself and other secondary features such as the attractive and appetising images on the product packaging. In this last respect, the artwork and graphics used is systematically designed and tested for maximum impact among the chosen target market. In fact, most of us would be amazed at the degree of care taken by large manufacturers in designing and testing every packaging detail, including labels and photos, to maximise our desire to consume a particular food. However, not all companies have the wherewithal to do this, as smaller manufacturers normally have to address other factors of competitiveness.

A good example of just how sophisticated this particular discipline has become are the breakfast cereal boxes of the larger companies of the sector. Not only is the product inside made to look incredibly appetising (even though it often really looks nothing like that) but the selection of colours is also meticulously thought out. Have you ever noticed that boxes of children's cereals always feature some kind of big-eyed funny character (normally an animal) looking downwards? This is no coincidence - the whim or preference of a cartoonist or a designer – but a direct consequence of the fact that this type of illustration has been proved to be very effective in attracting children's attention and in making them think that these characters are smiling down on them and inviting them to play.

Product positioning in food retailers is another aspect which has been carefully planned and studied. The most desirable products, those which we instinctively go for without thinking and frequently consume more out of pleasure than need, are normally to be found in pride of place in shops and on the shelves. Furthermore, as these are very often the manufacturers' most profitable products, they are also strategically placed for easy consumer access in the most frequently used aisles and at a convenient height. These are the most "valuable" areas in food retailers, those which give them their biggest profit margins. Even though we may have no intention of doing so, there's a good chance we'll end up there and let our most basic instincts get the better of us by falling victim to their "magnetism" and buying them.

It's therefore no surprise that product organisation in the most professional food retailers is now managed in a systematic and structured manner. Every shelf and aisle is segmented and classified to offer manufacturers the option which best meets their objectives in line with their available resources. But marketing experts do not only connect with our irrational and impulsive side; they also pay considerable attention to the more rational part of our brain, that part associated especially with the frontal cortex and generally with thinking and reasoning. That same part which in some cases will fight against our instinct to buy certain foods we know to be more rewarding but which, at the same time, we know to be not so good for our health.

In this case, the degree of marketing sophistication in its efforts to win over our more rational side is, once again, truly amazing. This time, marketing professionals hone in on two very powerful ideas which are also used in other fields: improved health and physical appearance. The basic messages used to ensure that the thinking and reasoning process undertaken in our frontal cortex reaches a clear and favourable conclusion are straightforward: this or that food is better for our health and helps prevent this or that illness or ailment, or will help us to lose weight or, at least, to avoid being overweight. Or both. And all this combines with the more instinctive signals related to the reward circuit to eventually persuade us to buy that delicious – but also healthy and nutritious – foodstuff.

Or at least, that's what the theory would have us believe. There can be no doubt that the industry knows perfectly well what it's doing. The strategy it uses to con our most rational and objective side into believing what they want us to believe is focused on what can be called nutritionism. I use this term here to group together all those activities focused on identifying and disseminating the idea of the supposed goodness of certain nutrients and components of food, thereby giving them a starring role in highly processed foods. And at the same time, creating a powerful marketing weapon. For example, if study findings have associated the presence of a certain vitamin or mineral with an improved prognosis of a certain illness, or with a reduced risk of contracting a certain disease, then all that needs to be done to market a certain food as being "healthier" is to add a certain amount of that component to it.

The opposite tactic of negative comparison can also be used. In this case, prominence is given to the harmful nature of some food component or another and a "lifesaving" replacement is offered as a healthier option. For example, because some observational studies have associated a higher consumption of fats with a greater prevalence of cardiovascular disease, fats are presented as something negative and fat-free, or so-called "light", products are created. Or carbohydrates are promoted as a supposedly healthier substitute for fats.

The first of these strategies, that of adding certain components associated with potential benefits, has probably become one of the revenue streams of greatest interest for food manufacturers, to the point where a specific category of food products, so-called "functional

148

foods", has been created around this idea. Current regulations permit the use of this term for those foods considered to have a potentially positive effect on health beyond basic nutrition.

The success of this type of product has forced officialdom into fast-tracking regulation of the use of corresponding health claims. However, as is often the case, the food industry reacts faster than officialdom, appearing to be permanently one step ahead of the rule makers. New terms, statements or words appear every now and then in the market which, despite their vagueness and without transgressing the law, dupe our brain into relating them with something positive and healthy. *"Strengthens your defences"*, *"Helps build strong and healthy bones"*, *"The strength you need"*, *"Improves intestinal transit"*... all these are advertising slogans carefully designed to appeal to the particular target audience of a product. A target audience which, though a little sceptical, is also looking to assuage its own particular health concerns.

These word games of dubious legality are often rooted in exaggerated claims and even stray into the domain of misleading publicity, which may end up in the courts. This, however, is not generally a difficult obstacle to overcome for the companies involved, as the law regulating this area of the business is quite lax and the issue can usually be resolved quite quickly with minor adjustments to their strategy.

And all this despite the fact that there has never been any proof that any product within this range of foodstuffs is genuinely useful for improving your health. Yes, that's right, you've read correctly. Not one study has ever provided unequivocal evidence of clear health benefits over and above the results gleaned from the conventional intermediate indicators used in these cases. In other words, there is no firm evidence of what specific illnesses are combated or of the extent to which mortality is reduced by consuming one or another of these functional foods.

To cap it all, existing regulations permit claims to be made in relation to specific isolated components, such as *"taken in the correct quantity, this*

micronutrient is associated with lower rates of such-and-such disease".
Under this legislation, manufacturers are under no obligation to clarify
that a banana or a steak may provide us with a much larger quantity of
this micronutrient, as well as a host of other nutrients, probably in a
tastier way and at a far lower cost. And neither are they under any
obligation to inform us of other less favourable components in their
products which could possibly even counteract their own health claim.

For example, dairy products with added calcium is an argument that
sells well, especially among women of a certain age group at risk of
osteoporosis. A lack of calcium has been associated with a greater risk
of osteoporosis, but that doesn't mean that this disease can effectively
be prevented by taking calcium-rich food supplements (normally dairy
products). Osteoporosis is caused by several factors, some of which are
still unknown to us, but we do know for a fact that excess calcium may
increase risk of coronary disease. Furthermore, many of these dairy
products with added calcium are rich in sugar, the effect of which on
our health may be less than favourable, particularly for overweight
people.

In any case, all you have to do to see the effect brought about by this
new food business is to take a look around your local supermarket and
compare the health claims attributed to the foods on display in different
areas and aisles. Some experts have actually done this on a systematic
basis, and the findings of their research are revealing. Paradoxically,
fresh foods, those which studies repeatedly associate with a longer life
and better health, carry practically no health claims. Vegetables, fruit,
meat and fish are displayed "no frills", or at most, with their price and
place of origin. Packaged foods with limited processing, such as pulses,
nuts, canned foods and frozen fresh fish and vegetables, also associated
with a healthy lifestyle, are put on display with information on their
nutritional composition and little more. Conversely, the areas displaying
functional foods, especially cereals, biscuits and complex dairy
products, are absolutely full of messages, images and cues suggesting
they are good for our health.

Confronted with this scenario and these tactics of persuasion, our brain has everything to lose. For thousands of millions of years, it has been shaped through evolutionary pressure to be especially sensitive, ingenious and resourceful in the face of food-related cues. As we've seen in other sections of this book, our irrational side is dominated by instinct and reacts to basic cues such as seeing and remembering food, which in turn activates the neurons of the reward circuit and floods them with dopamine, bringing about that intense and uncontrollable urge or sense of desire. At the same time, the most rational or thoughtful side of our brain is conveniently "reprogrammed" by extremely persuasive messages, ideas and associations, all dressed up as rigour and science and suggesting benefits both for our health and/or our physical appearance.

In this case, the two perspectives converge with no way back, leading us to take the decision the food industry most hopes for and desires: to buy and consume their products.

Children, the weakest link

This situation is further compounded by the perverse use of food advertising aimed at children. As with adults, a child's brain is sensitive to the most primary sensory signals, particularly those associated with sweet things, anticipating pleasure and reward when faced with delicious-looking and crispy sugary foods. However, the rational perspective of a child's brain is very different to that of an adult. In this case, the notion of a "healthy eating habit", something of a clearly long-term preventive nature requiring behavioural decisions to be taken in the present, doesn't really come into play or make much sense. A child's brain is simply not prepared for this set of concepts. As all parents know, the long-term perspective is something we develop as we mature, and it's practically impossible to convince a child of something by speaking of future possibilities.

For this very reason, industrial psychology and marketing experts use a different approach with children to strengthen the homeostatic and hedonic drive triggered by their attractive-looking products. In this case, advertising messages focus on another type of benefit adapted to the world of children and related to their need to play and have fun. The best-known and most conspicuous technique is to give away toys, picture cards or some other gimmick with the product, but there are other more commonplace practices designed to penetrate deep into the cerebral cortex. As mentioned above, colourful cartoon characters, often friendly-looking and cuddly animals, are depicted on the packaging looking down towards children. These characters are always happy-looking and full of energy, and are often portrayed as being particularly good at some sport or another or having some kind of special powers after eating the magical ingredients of the foodstuff in question. In short, a great taste in a happy and fun environment.

But there's more. The power and sophistication of children's food marketing is truly impressive. Food companies hire the most creative professionals in the market and the best designers and animators for advertising campaigns characterised by repetitive but highly child-friendly messages, especially aimed at prime-time children's TV and videogames. Children's programmes, with their continual commercial breaks and covert sponsors, have become extremely profitable for TV channels, with the added bonus that the broadcasters receive no complaints about this as the adverts are usually considered by children to be more entertaining and more fun than the programmes themselves.

Advertising standards don't help much either. Though regulatory criteria have been established in many countries, food advertisers have most commonly adopted a programme of self-regulation, and strict compliance with such regulation is not particularly high on their agenda. At the end of the day, who's going to take them to task on this issue? The grim reality of the matter is that advertising brings in money, and without money, there's no television.

Children are not capable of understanding that all this is nothing more than a strategy to persuade them to do something. The concept of inhibiting or repressing their impulse to eat something is practically non-existent in their brain, as they are driven primarily by senses such as flavour, appearance, smell and positive reinforcement. With this in mind, it's easy to imagine just how vulnerable children are to this bombardment of emotional cues, the objective of which is not to improve their welfare or health but simple to sell more products. Food products. And not, by chance, vegetables, fruit or fresh food, but breakfast cereals, pastries, sweets and sugary drinks.

This situation is of great concern. Nowadays, the food on sale for our children is nutritionally inferior to the food on sale for us adults. Most of this food has an extremely high sugar content and tastes sweet, and sweetness is the first taste that a baby's brain is capable of discerning and detecting. This same taste is what continually triggers the baby's reward circuit. If sweetness is predominant in everything the child eats during his/her infancy, it will end up becoming essential every time he or she eats something.

TV is by no means the only medium used by the marketing industry for child-targeted advertising. Sponsoring various types of child-focused activities is an especially attractive option, as it provides sponsors with a magnificent opportunity to showcase their products and brands by associating them with something children like and think is fun.

However, the practice I find the most perverse of all and which riles me the most is the one that masquerades under the slogan "health campaign". Usually fronted by some kind of association or foundation but funded, behind the scenes, by a food company, these initiatives typically hire unscrupulous members of the healthcare sector to endorse their argument, and incompetent politicians to secure media coverage and the required permission to present what they have to offer in schools. Both collectives, of course, are frequently "compensated" accordingly for their efforts. Talks, leaflets, posters, websites and freebies are then used in schools to attract and ensnare children, parents and teachers alike. Though disguised as some kind of event in the interest of society, the only real purpose of these "health campaigns" is to embed, in the most rational area of the brain of their target audience, all the messages required for them to choose a specific company's products when shopping for their children's and their own breakfast, lunch and afternoon snack.

If any such campaign is launched in your children's school under the title of "a healthy breakfast" or "a balanced afternoon snack", I recommend you look into it a bit further. You may well find there's a business or manufacturer behind it aiming to wangle their products into the school by using unsubstantiated claims, myths or studies conveniently interpreted to suit their interests. Products which are nearly always unhealthy and a million miles from fruit, vegetables and fresh food.

I urge you to report these practices to the relevant authorities.

REFERENCES

Alimentación y desarrollo encefálico en la evolución del linaje humano (Perez-Iglesias JI, 2012)

Metabolic constraint imposes tradeoff between body size and number of brain neurons in human evolution (Fonseca-Azevedo et al, 2012)

Proximity of foods in a competitive food environment influences consumption of a low calorie and a high calorie food (Privitera et al, 2014)

Salt Sugar Fat: How the Food Giants Hooked Us (Michael Moss, 2013)

Eating beyond metabolic need: how environmental cues influence feeding behabior (Johnson, 2013)

Food marketing targeting youth and families: what do we know about stores where moms actually shop? (Rooney et al, 2014)

The effects of food advertising and cognitive load on food choices (Zimmerman, 2014)

Eyes in the Aisles: Why Is Cap'n Crunch Looking Down at My Child? (Wansink et al, 2014)

A systematic review of persuasive marketing techniques to promote food to children on television (Jenkin et al, 2014)

Art of persuasion: an analysis of techniques used to market foods to children (Hebden et al, 2011)

The influence of the Children's Food and Beverage Advertising Initiative: change in children's exposure to food advertising on television in Canada between 2006-2009 (Potvin et al, 2014)

'I saw Santa drinking soda!' Advertising and children's food preferences (Lioutas et al, 2014)

Evaluation of food and beverage television advertising during children's viewing time in Spain using the UK nutrient profile model (Romero-Fernandez et al, 2013)

Influence of food companies' brand mascots and entertainment companies' cartoon media characters on children's diet and health: a systematic review and research needs (Kraak y otros)

Marketing foods to children: a comparison of nutrient content between children's and non-children's products (2014)

Evaluating Industry Self-Regulation of Food Marketing to Children (Kunkel et al, 2015)

Sugar as part of a balanced breakfast? What cereal advertisements teach children about healthy eating (LoDolce et al, 2013)

Food and beverage advertising during children's television programming (Scully et al, 2014)

Influence of Spanish TV commercials on child obesity (2015)

Evaluating Industry Self-Regulation of Food Marketing to Children (Kunkel et al, 2015)

PART 3

REPROGRAMMING THE BRAIN

Before putting forward some ideas and solutions to address many of the issues discussed in this book, I'd like to be completely honest with you and make one thing crystal clear. As I have said on many occasions in previous chapters, many of the hypotheses and theories referred to in this book are still at a fledgling stage of development. Though important discoveries are being made, the hypotheses proposed to date are, as yet, not particularly sound, and there is still a lot of work to be done regarding in-depth research into the relation between the brain and being overweight. It therefore follows that whilst this is the case, great care must be taken with proposals for real practical treatment.

The truth of the matter is that very few clinical trials designed from neurological and psychological perspectives have produced encouraging results in connection with the battle against obesity. In fact, in certain subject areas, hardly any trials have been conducted. The recommendations that follow in this part of the book are, therefore, guarded, but made on the basis of conclusions drawn from numerous scientific studies. Consequently, these recommendations will tend to be of a generic and conservative nature.

And please remember: it's always a good idea to maintain a healthy degree of scepticism and critical awareness.

3.1. FIXING THE "THERMOSTAT"

Having looked at the numerous lifestyle and habit-related environmental variables which may imbalance our brain and cause operational problems, perhaps the most reasonable thing now is to start identifying those habits we should change if we want to return the biochemical and metabolic machinery that regulates our energy intake to a normal state of being.

The first thing to do is to focus on the systems controlling energy homeostasis, particularly the nervous sensors and key hormones, and on the processes related to the reward circuit. Having said that, I would once again like to point out that there is no firm evidence of the existence of various types of clearly differentiated food intake (such as homeostatic and hedonic): nevertheless, I shall occasionally continue to use this classification, as I consider it useful from a didactic point of view to explain certain ideas more clearly.

So, taking all these considerations into account, for the first chapter of this section I have drawn up ten guidelines on eating and psychosocial habits to help you correct the causes and the origin of the problems discussed in previous sections of this book. Some of these guidelines are more evidence-based than others but, irrespective of this, the advice and recommendations put forward here are all potentially useful and will certainly do you no harm at all. In fact, they're very likely to do you good. One or two of them may appear to be a little vague but unfortunately, for the moment, it's not really possible in those cases for me to be any more specific given the current state of scientific knowledge. In any case, I believe it best to leave the details in each case to the experts and specialists in these matters, who are in a better position to adapt and customise the actions that need to be taken to the end objective and personal circumstances of each individual. For example, dietary issues should be specifically addressed by dieticians, psychosocial issues by psychologists, and exercise-related issues by trainers or fitness coaches. Each individual and each case is different, so the priority to be given to each of these guidelines will vary and needs to be customised accordingly.

So, here is a 10-point-plan for reprogramming the brain.

1. Help your hypothalamus and digestive sensors to do their job well

There are several habits and conditioning factors which contribute to helping the orexigenic and anorexigenic neurons of the hypothalamus receive the signals arriving from the different organs of our body and, consequently, to perform as hunger switches, triggering, as appropriate, feelings of hunger or of being full. One of these factors is time.

If you give importance both to what you eat and to eating itself, and you set aside for them the time and attention they deserve, then you'll be helping your hypothalamus to do its job properly. Findings from many studies link eating calmly and chewing food thoroughly with a lower body weight. By doing so, the required hormones have more time to be secreted (these hormones are not secreted immediately) and a better chance of reaching their neuronal receptors.

You may also remember from a previous chapter of this book that the reason why obese people derive less pleasure from eating is probably because their neurons have grown accustomed to very intense and pleasurable tastes and have, so to speak, become desensitised. To compensate for this, it's advisable to concentrate on making an effort to enjoy the act of eating itself: looking at the food, being aware of its smell and its texture in your mouth and getting the most out of its taste. This will help you obtain the same sense of satisfaction as always but eating smaller quantities of food, and you may even manage to increase the pleasure you get from eating fresh food which has not been industrially processed to make it more palatable.

Another recommendation here is to avoid eating whilst doing some other intellectually complex activity or something that requires you to think, like watching TV, for example. In recent times, this has become an increasingly common and bad habit amongst children when sitting at the meal table. In these cases, our prefrontal cortex, the part of the brain which takes charge of thinking and planning, becomes distracted with things other than what is really important, i.e. our nutrition, thereby exposing us to the risk of losing a certain amount of control and, almost without realising, eating too much. Furthermore, this bad practice distracts our brain from concentrating on and appreciating the potentially gratifying sensations of less palatable foods, as its attention will be focused on the screen instead of on the act of eating.

Not eating highly processed foods will also be positive for your hypothalamus. This is especially so if these foods have been manufactured using ultra-refined ingredients and have undergone radical processes of transformation and/or have been pre-cooked, as this will have made them highly digestible. When consumed, these foods are absorbed very quickly and efficiently, giving our digestive sensors very little time to detect them and to release enough of the hormones and signals required. In this respect, it is much better for us to eat those foods which our digestive system has to work a little harder on. Try to ensure your diet is mostly made up of fresh produce, fundamentally a wide variety of vegetables, providing plenty of fibre (which slows down food absorption), as well as fresh fish, meat and eggs. These may be supplemented by pulses and nuts, a much better source of nutrients and less easy to digest than cereal products.

Be careful with your protein intake from this fresh produce. As a micronutrient, a minimum amount of protein should be consumed to ensure availability of the necessary amino acids and to take advantage of its satiating power (protein is considered to be the most satiating macronutrient). This does *not* mean you should stuff yourself eating proteins or that you will lose weight by cramming them into your diet, but study findings reveal that it's recommendable to ensure a reasonable protein intake to avoid a loss of muscle mass when losing weight and to help us feel full. The recommended amount is 1-1.5g pure protein per day/ kilogram of body weight. In other words, if you weigh 100 kilos, it would be recommendable for you to eat 100-150g protein per day. But be careful... I'm talking about proteins, not foods. You'll have to calculate the amount of food you need to obtain the amount of proteins required (for example, you'll need around 400-500g of fish to obtain 100g protein).

I'll end the first of these recommended guidelines by reminding you that another way to help your stomach duly send out the desired satiety signals is by drinking water. Making a habit of hydrating before eating not only slakes your thirst (being thirsty may also generate a certain level of anxiety) but also contributes to filling your stomach, which means you'll need to eat less food to reach that point of feeling full when the corresponding signals are channelled through to the brain.

2. Keep your glucose and insulin levels under control

When it comes to the best approach for managing insulin and glucose, study findings are clear. The key is firstly to prevent hyperinsulinemia, characterised, as we've seen in previous sections of this book, by high levels of glucose in the blood and sudden and chronic fluctuations of this condition, and secondly, to avoid high blood triglyceride levels. This latter factor, you may also remember, may be the cause of insulin resistance, as it impedes the passage of insulin through the blood-brain barrier.

From a dietary point of view, the best way to achieve this (to keep glucose and insulin levels under control and to ensure low blood triglyceride levels) is to eat less highly processed, fast-digesting and carbohydrate-rich foodstuffs (pastries, biscuits, snacks, breakfast cereals, bread, potatoes, rice, sugary drinks, etc.) and more slow-digesting carbohydrates with a high fibre content (vegetables, fruits and pulses). Another possibility is to opt for whole grain versions of the less desirable foods listed in the previous sentence. However, this option has its drawbacks, as the lack of specific legislation in this area means that certain products marketed as whole grain are essentially questionable as such. In any case, when faced with the choice, it is much better to choose a vegetable or even a pulse dish as the main course of a meal.

3. Prevent leptin resistance and chronically high concentrations of this hormone

Though hypotheses on the cause of leptin resistance require further research and proof, there is sufficient evidence to suspect that it is expedited by excess sugars and chronically high levels of insulin.

The recommendation, therefore, is clear and specific: avoid foods with a high added sugar content, especially if they also contain refined carbohydrates: for example, sugared drinks, sweets, pastries, biscuits, breakfast cereals, juices and milk products containing added sugar, amongst others.

4. Avoid chronic or systemic inflammation

Prevention of chronic inflammation is of key importance, as the components secreted by our organism to combat it have a negative effect on the correct functioning and balance of the "energy regulator" controlled by our brain. It's also likely that chronic inflammation is involved in developing resistance to certain hormones. However, in this particular case, it's not so easy to give exact instructions as to how to avoid it, as inflammation is an enormously complex phenomenon which can be brought on by many different situations and habits.

There are also reasonable grounds to believe that exercise may help to reduce inflammation. From a dietary perspective, the main culprits would once again seem to be highly processed foods, especially those high in fats, salt, sugars and calories, as avoiding these foods normally reduces the levels of corresponding inflammatory markers. Furthermore, processed meats (cold and sausage meats), foods cooked at very high temperatures (with food degradation and/or oil) and trans fats are all associated with an increase in inflammatory cytokines. Conversely, eating fibre-rich fresh food generally reduces the concentration of some of these cytokines.

In any case, as obesity itself is the main factor in exacerbating inflammation, the basic recommendation in this case is to focus your efforts on keeping your weight down to a reasonable level.

5. *Rewire your reward circuit*

Though there is still a certain amount of controversy surrounding this issue, it appears quite plausible that if highly palatable foods (those which trigger an acute response from the reward system) are regularly consumed in high quantities over a number of years, our brain progressively becomes accustomed to those intense flavours and sensations. One consequence of this reduced sensitivity is that fresh and natural food may lose its appeal and be considered as less enjoyable and desirable. At the same time, increasingly more intense flavours are required to maintain the same degree of enjoyment, so we end up needing to consume ever more palatable and pleasurable foods. The end result is a never-ending vicious circle which gets worse over time.

Obviously, the first thing to do to prevent this from happening is to put a stop to the downward spiral. The only way to do this is to minimise your consumption of highly processed and flavoured foods. Generally speaking, these foods are high in fats, salt, sugar and refined carbohydrates, and have a very high calorie content. Once again, I'm mainly referring to all foods derived from cereals and potatoes (pastries, bread, cakes, biscuits, breakfast cereals, snacks, crisps, etc.), pre-cooked foods (pizza, deep-fried foods, etc.) and those with a high sugar content (sugared drinks, ice-cream, etc.).

And what does "minimise" mean? None at all? A lot less? Well, the only answer I can give is "it depends", as everything *will* depend on how your brain reacts to these foods and on the amount of them involved. Physiologically, none of the foods mentioned in the paragraph above are necessary to stay healthy (just the opposite, in fact), so you wouldn't become any less healthy by not eating any of them. Likewise, it's also true that there are many different foods in that list and that many people have no problem eating them in reasonable amounts. What

I can say categorically is that they should not form the basis of your diet but be eaten occasionally.

To get a better idea of your own personal situation, try first to identify exactly which foods you are most likely to lose control over and have a craving for. Then, try different strategies to eat less of them, reducing the amount more or less and/or eating them less often. For example, try eating small amounts every day, or just once a week but a larger amount. Be aware of how your brain responds to these changes, but never lose sight of the need to avoid situations in which you are likely to lose control and binge eat these foods.

The key is to remain as rational as possible about all this and not to allow yourself to be overcome by an emotional response, such as feeling guilty about a lax moment in which you succumb to eating more than you had planned to. Study findings show that this type of reaction is counterproductive. Just file it under "lessons learnt" and continue as normal with your life, devising a strategy to ensure a balance between minimising the intake of these foods and the satisfaction they give you.

Another good idea is to remember at all times what experts have found when analysing the brain activity of obese people. Allow me to remind you: findings have revealed that the response, in obese people, of the reward circuit to images and other such cues of highly palatable food generates exaggerated expectations and large-scale secretion of dopamine, which in turn spurs them on to take the decision to look for and consume those foods. This behaviour is then wrongly interpreted by many people as a lack of willpower. So, don't put yourself in situations which may cause this type of problem for you. For example, stay away from those areas of the supermarket where these foods are on display, especially if you haven't eaten for a while, and avoid those occasions (such as buffet meals) when it's very difficult to choose something to eat without feasting your eyes on the most appetising but least recommendable dishes. You'd also be well advised, especially if children are involved, to keep well away from those brightly-coloured and attention-seeking sweet vending machines, and it goes without saying that it's not a good idea to have a secret stack of this type of food stashed away in a cupboard at home "to pick at now and again" or "in case we have visitors".

However, rewiring your reward circuit is not just a case of limiting your consumption of those foods which overstimulate it. You can also try to reprogramme it by increasing its sensitivity to healthier foods. In this case, the idea is to acclimatise the brain back to appreciating the value of those healthier foods which can also be rewarding for you. In this respect, reducing your intake of highly palatable foods is likely to increase the sensitivity of the brain's reward area and to return its receptors to normal, thereby enabling you to savour the sensory subtleties and virtues of fresh produce. This is exactly what happens to those people who radically reduce their intake of sugar and highly sweetened foods over a period of time: when they eat a piece of cake or drink a sugary drink some time later, it tastes sickly sweet to them. So much so that, in some cases, they opt for a piece of fresh fruit instead. And it's a similar story with ex-smokers who, having given up smoking some time ago, take a drag on a cigarette. The result? What before gave them pleasure now tastes awful.

There are, additionally, several other things you can do on a proactive basis to streamline this process of reprogramming in favour of healthy foods. One way is to give healthy eating a more prominent role in your life by dedicating more time and energy to it and managing it in a constructive, interesting and fun way. For example, when you go shopping, take time and care in choosing fresh ingredients, and explore new ideas for preparing, cooking and presenting them. And why not share your food with family and friends (when was the last time you sat down for a quiet dinner with your family?), making meal time a pleasant and enjoyable experience.

All this will help your brain to once again create expectations around these foods, include them amongst its priorities, revalue them and enable you to give them their due worth. And little by little, you'll discover that eating these foods can also give you pleasure, the right and necessary type of pleasure, no more and no less, and with no side effects.

6. Don't critically disrupt your circadian rhythms

In this case, the advice is simple: sleep as much as you need to feel refreshed, and if possible, avoid abrupt and frequent changes in your sleep schedule. And sleep with the light off. There's no need for bright lights at home at night, and in any case, keeping lights on is expensive and not at all sustainable.

Another good idea is to take a few minutes whenever you can to soak up the sun during the day (but be careful not to burn yourself!). If you can turn this into a daily habit, so much the better. This not only affords your brain and the rest of your metabolism exposure to sunlight but also enables vitamin D to be produced in your body. Vitamin D deficiency is associated with many health problems.

7. Look after your microbiota and your microbiota will look after you

Remember there's a large family of intestinal microbes inside you that you need to keep in good health: if you look after them, they'll look after you. There are two strategies involved here: the first is to avoid eating those foods that they don't particularly "like" and may even be harmful for them (the usual suspects: processed and palatable foods high in fats, salt, sugar and refined carbohydrates, and processed meats), and the second is to give priority to the foods they most "like", such as fibre-rich vegetables, fruits and pulses and fermented milk products such as natural yogurt.

Finally, only take antibiotics on doctor's orders, as these drugs destroy a lot of your intestinal residents.

8. Be sceptical and critical about food marketing

I'll say it again, loud and clear, to make sure you get the message: the primary objective of food companies is to sell. This means that anything and everything they tell you is likely to be biased towards this end objective, which is not necessarily the same as yours, i.e. to look after your health. This being so, it's just not worth taking the risk of being persuaded this way, especially when confronted with people with such sophisticated powers of persuasion as the marketing experts of the big corporations.

Ignore, or even better, avoid those advertisements on food and health and the promises they make. Forget about functional and supplementary foods unless recommended or prescribed by your doctor or dietician. If your diet is made up of fresh and healthy food, you normally won't need them anyway.

Be especially careful about this with children, and don't leave them to take their own decisions on what they eat, particularly if those decisions are influenced by publicity. Children are not capable of distinguishing between what's healthy and what isn't... what they'll ask for is what they most like or takes their fancy. In this respect, what *you* must do is provide them with healthy food and act as a role-model by eating those same foods with them. And don't resort to food to compensate for certain problems, to convince children to do something or as a reward to stop complaining or crying. Food is there for us to feed ourselves... end of story.

9. Minimise stress

As discussed in a previous section of this book, stress is another variable which exacerbates many of the imbalances caused by bad habits. Stress is associated, amongst other things, with a resistance to certain hormones, with inflammation, with imbalances in our sleep schedule and our microbiota and with the need to compensate for distress by eating highly palatable foods (emotional eating). The need to manage and minimise stress as much as possible is, therefore, obvious.

Having said this, I am not so naive as to think that a problem as complex as stress can be solved with a few simple pieces of advice.

Nowadays, stress is an enormous challenge for psychologists, so I will simply limit myself here to listing some possible origins of stress in the hope that this may be a first step towards solving this problem for you.

According to the findings of a survey conducted in 2014, the main sources of stress for people in North America are, in decreasing order of importance, as follows:

- Too many responsibilities

- Money

- Work

- My own health problems

- Health problems affecting members of my family

- Members of my family

- Personal appearance

I recommend you give some thought to whether the stress you're suffering is rooted in any of these sources. If it is, my recommendation would be to start thinking about how to put a stop to those sources. I know it's not easy but you have to start somewhere.

10. Keep active and do exercise

If you thought your brain was going to be exempt from this guideline, think again! It is absolutely essential to avoid a sedentary lifestyle and to do physical exercise. In this case, I'm not going to justify this statement by trotting out the normal argument that exercise burns calories, as our body generally compensates for this by consequently making us feel hungry. And neither do you need me to remind you of the proven benefits of regular exercise for your health, especially with respect to helping prevent cardiovascular disease, to considerably prolonging your physical fitness and self-sufficiency and to increasing your life expectation. I take it for granted you are aware of this already.

However, within the context of what's under discussion in this book, what you *do* need to know is that exercise is associated with reduced insulin and leptin resistance and reduced systemic inflammation, both of which, as you will remember, are factors provoking an imbalance in our brain, our energy regulator. Furthermore, exercise is highly effective in combating stress and depression, as it triggers the release of neurotransmitters such as serotonin which make us feel better and more energetic. And exercise doesn't only *prevent* problems: many studies have shown that physical activity significantly improves the performance of the brain, both in a general cognitive sense and particularly with respect to memory. Some studies even suggest that it could even improve the plasticity, or flexibility, of the brain. So, it would be fair to say that physical exercise not only helps develop the muscles in your body but also in your brain.

Additionally, evidence from (a relatively few) studies undertaken on the subject to date suggests that intense physical exercise may be useful in attempting to reprogramme our brain (as addressed above in the fifth guideline). Some research has shown that doing sport may reduce the desire to eat less recommendable (highly palatable and high-calorie) foods, and increase our expectations for, and the value we give to, healthier (and generally less caloric) foods.

And to finish, the best exercise for you to do is the one you like most and can keep doing over time. In any case, if you're interested in this issue, study findings show that the ideal situation is to combine two types of activity: aerobic exercise (running, cycling, football, tennis, dancing, etc.) and anaerobic exercise (weights, strength exercises, etc.).

A summary of the habits included in the 10 guidelines:

1. *Help your hypothalamus and digestive sensors to do their job well.*

2. *Keep your glucose and insulin levels under control.*

3. *Prevent leptin resistance and chronically high concentrations of this hormone.*

4. *Avoid chronic or systemic inflammation.*

5. *Rewire your reward circuit.*

6. *Don't critically disrupt your circadian rhythms.*

7. *Look after your microbiota.*

8. *Be sceptical and critical about food marketing.*

9. *Minimise stress.*

10. *Keep active and do exercise.*

A chart is included on the next page to accompany this 10-point-plan. This food pyramid, taken from my book entitled "What science tells us about losing weight", provides a visual reference as to how to prioritise one of the most important aspects of this plan: the food to eat. This may prove useful for you in your attempts to follow the different dietary recommendations included in the plan.

ORIENTATIVE PORTIONS OF EACH FOOD GROUP

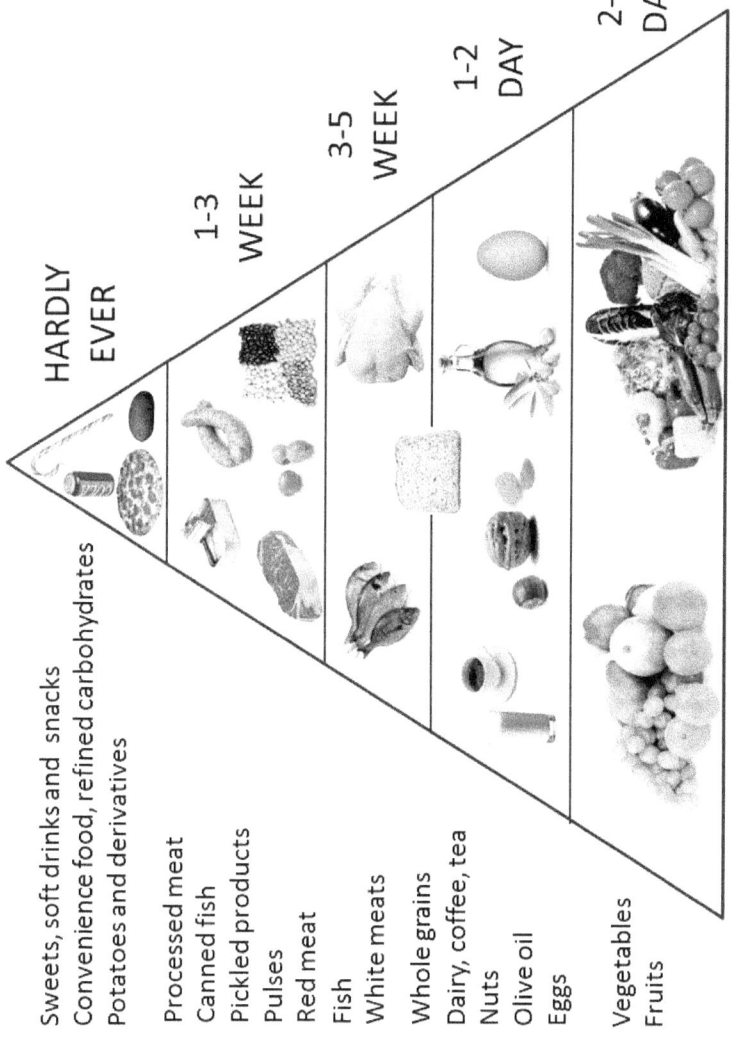

HARDLY EVER — Sweets, soft drinks and snacks; Convenience food, refined carbohydrates; Potatoes and derivatives

1-3 WEEK — Processed meat; Canned fish; Pickled products; Pulses; Red meat

3-5 WEEK — Fish; White meats

1-2 DAY — Whole grains; Dairy, coffee, tea; Nuts; Olive oil; Eggs

2-4 DAY — Vegetables; Fruits

REFERENCES

Eating 'attentively' reduces later energy consumption in overweight and obese females (Robinson et al, 2014)

Eating slowly increases the postprandial response of the anorexigenic gut hormones, peptide YY and glucagon-like peptide-1 (Kokkinos et al, 2010)

Mindfulness-based interventions for obesity-related eating behaviours: a literature review (O'Reilly et al, 2014)

Mindfulness meditation as an intervention for binge eating, emotional eating, and weight loss: a systematic review (Katterman, 2014)

Dealing with problematic eating behaviour. The effects of a mindfulness-based intervention on eating behaviour, food cravings, dichotomous thinking and body image concern (Alberts et al, 2012)

Attention with a mindful attitude attenuates subjective appetitive reactions and food intake following food-cue exposure (2015)

Metabolic benefits of dietary prebiotics in human subjects: a systematic review of randomised controlled trials (Kellow y otro, 2014)

Effects of dietary fibre on subjective appetite, energy intake and body weight: a systematic review of randomized controlled trials (Wanders, 2011)

The short-chain fatty acid acetate reduces appetite via a central homeostatic mechanism (Bell et al, 2014)

High protein intake stimulates postprandial GLP1 and PYY release (Klaauw, et al, 2013)

Increased Carbohydrate Induced Ghrelin Secretion in Obese vs. Normal-weight Adolescent Girls (Misra et al, 2009)

Comparison of postprandial profiles of ghrelin, active GLP-1, and total PYY to meals varying in fat and carbohydrate and their association with hunger and the phases of satiety (Gibbons et al, 2013)

Successful weight loss maintenance includes long-term increased meal responses of GLP-1 and PYY 3-36 (2016)

Association between water consumption and body weight outcomes: a systematic review (Muckelbauer R et al, 2013)

Association of fructose consumption and components of metabolic síndrome in human studies: A systematic review and meta-analysis (Kelishadi, 2013)

Long-term effects of low glycemic index/load vs. high glycemic index/load diets on parameters of obesity and obesity-associated risks: a systematic review and meta-analysis (Schwingshackl et al, 2013)

Leptin Is Associated With Exaggerated Brain Reward and Emotion Responses to Food Images in Adolescent Obesity (Jastreboff et al, 2014)

Effect of dietary fiber on circulating C-reactive protein in overweight and obese adults: a meta-analysis of randomized controlled trials (Jiao et al, 2015)

Dietary factors affect food reward and motivation to eat (Pandit, 2012)

Nutritional Controls of Food Reward (Fernandes et al, 2015)

Proximity of foods in a competitive food environment influences consumption of a low calorie and a high calorie food (Privitera, 2014)

Impact of the removal of chocolate milk from school milk programs for children in Saskatoon, Canada (Henry et al, 2015)

Excessive Sugar Consumption May Be a Difficult Habit to Break: A View From the Brain and Body (Tryon et al, 2015)

Recent studies of the effects of sugars on brain systems involved in energy balance and reward: Relevance to low calorie sweeteners (2016)

Reduced dietary intake of simple sugars alters perceived sweet taste intensity but not perceived pleasantness (2015)

How palatable food disrupts appetite regulation (Erlanson, 2005)

Effects of dietary glycemic index on brain regions related to reward and craving in men (2013)

Neural systems underlying the reappraisal of personally craved foods (Giuliani, 2014)

Piece of cake. Cognitive reappraisal of food craving (Giuliano, 2013)

Pilot randomized trial demonstrating reversal of obesity-related abnormalities in reward system responsivity to food cues with a behavioral intervention (Deckersbach et al, 2014)

Brain response to food stimulation in obese, normal weight, and successful weight loss maintainers (Sweet et al, 2012)

"Restrained eating" vs "trying to lose weight": how are they associated with body weight and tendency to overeat among postmenopausal women? (Rideout et al, 2009)

Eating behavior correlates of adult weight gain and obesity in healthy women aged 55-65 y (Hays et al, 2002)

Chocolate cake. Guilt or celebration? Associations with healthy eating attitudes, perceived behavioural control, intentions and weight-loss (Kuijer et al, 2013)

Associating a prototypical forbidden food item with guilt or celebration: Relationships with indicators of (un)healthy eating and the moderating role of stress and depressive symptoms (Kuijer et al, 2014)

Is cooking at home associated with better diet quality or weight-loss intention? (Wolfson et al, 2014)

Is eating behavior manipulated by the gastrointestinal microbiota? Evolutionary pressures and potential mechanisms (Alcock et al, 2014)

Antibiotic use and childhood body mass index trajectory (2015)

The Burden of Stress in America (2014)

Associations between child emotional eating and general parenting style, feeding practices, and parent psychopathology (Braden et al, 2014)

Physical Activity and Cardiorespiratory Fitness Are Beneficial for White Matter in Low-Fit Older Adults (Burzinska et al, 2014)

Effects of exercise on gut peptides, energy intake and appetite (Martins, 2014)

Effects of exercise intensity on plasma concentrations of appetite-regulating hormones: Potential mechanisms (2015)

Effects of exercise of different intensity on gut peptides, energy intake and appetite in young males (Bilski et al, 2013)

Effects of different modes of exercise on appetite and appetite-regulating hormones (Kawano et al, 2013)

Impact of exercise training without caloric restriction on inflammation, insulin resistance and visceral fat mass in obese adolescents (Mendelson et al, 2014)

Inflammatory markers and adipocytokine responses to exercise training and detraining in men who are obese (Nikseresht et al, 2014)

Benefits of Regular Exercise on Inflammatory and Cardiovascular Risk Markers in Normal Weight, Overweight and Obese Adults (Gondim et al, 2015)

A single bout of resistance exercise can enhance episodic memory performance (Weinberg et al, 2014)

Exercise-induced noradrenergic activation enhances memory consolidation in both normal aging and patients with amnestic mild cognitive impairment (Segal et al, 2012)

A randomized controlled trial of multicomponent exercise in older adults with mild cognitive impairment (Suzuki et al, 2012)

Effects of an acute bout of exercise on memory in 6th grade children (Etnier et al, 2014)

Effects of exercise on anxiety and depression disorders: review of meta-analyses and neurobiological mechanisms (Wegner et al, 2014)

Physical exercise and brain responses to images of high-calorie food (Killgore, 2013)

The effects of high-intensity exercise on neural responses to images of food (crabtree, 2014)

The Power of the Mind: The Cortex as a Critical Determinant of Muscle Strength/Weakness (Clarck et al, 2014)

A cycling lane for brain rewiring (2015)

3.2. TREATING AN ADDICTION

The very idea of the existence of "food addiction" may well have been quite novel for you. If so, I'm not surprised, as this is not a commonly held perspective. The basic, widespread and oft-repeated premise for being overweight is an imbalance between the intake of calories and those which are expended by the body, which is vastly different to the concept of food addiction.

However, it is in no way a new idea; far from it, in fact. In the 1940s and 50s, a strong current of belief arose amongst psychiatrists in the United States of the need to convince society that obesity, just like alcoholism and problems with drugs, was rooted in an addiction, and that treating obesity could therefore be approached on this basis. Unfortunately, however, though these were times of great interest for researchers into the history of obesity, this idea came to an abrupt end when the previously mentioned model of energy imbalance (the combination of overeating and not doing enough exercise) unreservedly won the day and has prevailed ever since. It should also be said that, in terms of their scientific rigour and clinical outcomes, those early efforts at establishing the theory of eating addiction were a complete disaster. Firstly, the stigma attached to substance addiction was, at that time, enormous: the general view held of such addicts by society was that they were mostly idle and deceitful good-for-nothings and criminals. In those days, respect for the most disadvantaged members of society was at a premium, which didn't help the situation at all. All of which meant that this new proposal to consider overweight people as "addicts" served, more than anything else, to increase the likelihood of them being subject to even greater social contempt, as their possibilities of improving their situation were, to all intents and purposes, minimal.

Furthermore, the methods used by psychiatrists in those days to treat addictions could be described as pure pseudoscience. As we shall see in greater detail later on in this book, one of the major problems facing this specialist area of psychiatry in the modern day is the lack of scientific backing when attempting to develop effective treatments, so imagine what the situation was like over 50 years ago! Radical and absurd versions of Freudian theories were rampant, as were totally unsubstantiated practices and therapies, all of which in the end found some kind of psychoanalytical justification for blaming the patient (or their family) for everything and making them exclusively responsible for their problem.

To cap it all, certain unscrupulous pharmaceutical companies jumped on the bandwagon and took advantage to try to sell their most powerful drugs and antidepressants to long-suffering overweight people, promising to improve their mental state and, consequently, helping them to shed excess body fat. In all this, the least harmful treatment available to patients, and one that was chiefly promoted through the public health sector, was a type of group-based therapy involving psychoanalytical approaches. Though initially promising, this practice was eventually shown to be clearly ineffective in the long term.

In short, it wouldn't be unfair to say that the cure was worse than the disease.

Returning to the modern day and before continuing any further, I'd like to make it clear at this point that the priority is to continue researching into the potentiality of food addiction as a valid model for a partial explanation of the obesity epidemic. There is, as yet, no consensus on this issue, so we'll have to wait and see, but if experts do eventually coincide that this hypothesis may be useful for the design of effective strategies, most intervention approaches addressed to date will most likely have to be modified. And new therapies establishing how to translate all these new ideas into clinical practice will subsequently need to be developed.

I don't know how long we'll have to wait for this to happen, if it ever actually happens, but until then, we can only speculate on what would happen should this situation arise. For example, we can draw parallels with the type of treatments currently used to overcome substance addiction, treatments which are based on the most solid scientific evidence possible.

How addictions are treated

A word of warning: extreme care must be taken when conducting this kind of benchmarking exercise. In research terms, addiction treatment is, unfortunately, years behind other medical disciplines, and clinical practice in this area has, until only quite recently, been characterised by a lack of rigour and as a pseudoscience. A report published in 2012 by *The Center on Addiction and Substance Abuse* at Columbia University concluded that "*of those who do receive treatment, few receive anything that approximates evidence-based care*". This conclusion is of particular concern in countries such as the United States, with a very high rate of alcohol and drug addiction and with several thousand treatment centres spread across the country, most of them private and with operational policies subject to practically no control. In 2015, three years after publication of the Columbia University report, the Institute of Medicine (IoM) reported on the lack of rigorous backing and protocols based on scientific evidence in psychosocial interventions in treatment for substance abuse.

To give you an idea of what these reports are referring to, a broad outline of the typical structure of a treatment of this type is shown below. This is the exact scenario that has been in existence (and still is in many treatment centres) until very recently.

a) Treatments generally last around one month.

b) An inpatient approach is normally recommended: in other words, the patient is admitted into the treatment centre as an inmate for the duration of the treatment, though treatment may, in some cases, also be given on an outpatient basis.

c) Abstinence is mandatory: the consumption of any substance is totally prohibited. This is closely monitored by conducting objective tests, e.g. urine and blood tests.

d) The primary therapeutic model used is group therapy, though other methods are also used on a complementary basis depending on the case. Educational talks and sessions are also included.

e) The members of staff providing advice include reformed addicts.

f) In many treatment centres, the rehabilitation process is conducted within a context of spirituality. To give you an insight into what I mean by this, many treatment centres in North America (particularly those specialised in alcoholism) have for many years followed the 12 Steps method. These steps are as follows:

1. We admitted we were powerless over alcohol – that our lives had become unmanageable.

2. Came to believe that a Power greater than ourselves could restore us to sanity.

3. Made a decision to turn our will and our lives over to the care of God as we understood him.

4. Made a searching and fearless moral inventory of ourselves.

5. Admitted to God, to ourselves, and to another human being the exact nature of our wrongs.

6. Were entirely ready to have God remove all these defects of character.

7. Humbly asked him to remove our shortcomings.

8. Made a list of all persons we had harmed, and became willing to make amends to them all.

9. Made direct amends to such people wherever possible, except when to do so would injure them or others.

10. Continued to take personal inventory, and when we were wrong, promptly admitted it.

11. Sought through prayer and meditation to improve our conscious contact with God as we understood him, praying only for knowledge of His will for us and the power to carry that out.

12. Having had a spiritual experience as the result of these steps, we tried to carry this message to other alcoholics, and to practice these principles in all our affairs.

I think these "12 steps" are sufficiently self-explanatory for you to understand the need for further work to be done on a scientific approach to addiction treatment. Let's hope this is the case, though an Internet search will likely temper your optimism on this issue. If you take a quick look at what's available, you'll find private centres offering a range of treatments ranging from music therapy to acupuncture, hypnotherapy and Reiki.

It should also be acknowledged that responsibility for improving this situation does not rest entirely in the hands of the private sector. The meagre resources assigned by public administration and governments to this problem, generally in the form of mostly low-level programmes which approach this issue in a vastly different way from how most citizens see it, have not exactly been given with a "front-stage" profile. And this despite the fact that in some cases, the expenditure involved is considerable. One such example are campaigns against smoking, which exponentially increases the likelihood of respiratory diseases, cancer and mortality. The reason for this is clear: whether we're prepared to admit it or not, addiction, and more particularly, addicts, still suffer from considerable social stigma, and this same stigma clearly overlaps with the stigma attached to obesity and obese people.

What results have these programmes produced? Have they been effective? It's difficult to say. Firstly, they appear not to be essential. Some 20-80% of people who have suffered some kind of addiction in their life have got over it without resorting to these programmes (the wide variation in this percentage figure is attributable to the fact that results are very different depending on the type of substance involved and the degree of addiction). A large proportion of these people are also known to suffer relapses and require repeat treatment, which is generally the same as the original.

In any case, you do not need to be an expert in the subject to be surprised by certain features of these approaches, such as the lack of well-designed studies proving the effectiveness of each of these therapies, the use of staff with no specific or health training or spirituality as the key line of approach. Fortunately, an ever-increasing body of experts and scientists in this discipline has developed in recent years with a clear focus on the practice of evidence-based medicine. These people have begun to work with new and promising approaches. As a first step, they have recognised and publicised that many of the principles and dogmas followed and practised for many years were not evidence-based. To remedy this alarming situation, these same professionals are currently leading research to develop an exact branch of healthcare rooted in a list of therapies of proven effectiveness.

Though these dedicated professionals recognise there is still a lot to do in this area, new approaches have already appeared in scientific literature. Furthermore, the more scientific treatment centres have brought in new approaches to treatment, including changes and developments such as:

1. A variable length of treatment customised to each case (normally longer than the previously standard one-month period).

2. Prioritisation of outpatient treatment, reserving inpatient treatment only for the most serious and problematic cases.

3. A more flexible stage of detoxification, adapted to the patient's degree of addiction. An assessment of the seriousness and possible effects of withdrawal symptoms, greater consideration given to the

possible use of substitute drugs and substances, possible moderate and controlled consumption of other substances which do not produce symptoms of addiction, etc.

4. Prioritisation of individual and customised therapy over traditional group therapy (though a group dynamic is useful to offer individual therapy). Special care to be taken with the make-up of groups, i.e. not to group together patients with very different degrees of addiction.

5. Avoidance of any kind of activity designed to hold patients responsible for their problem and to tell them, in a simplified manner, how they should solve it (for example, informative and educational talks). Evidence has shown this to be useless and even counter-productive.

6. The exclusive use of professional and specialised health personnel, with the required training and specific competences.

7. The use of other therapeutic methods which, as well as helping and motivating patients to maintain their abstinence, support them in resolving emotional issues and other such problems of a psychological and social nature which may have arisen in conjunction with their addiction, e.g. family disorders, employment and financial needs, undesirable habits and/or relationships, etc.

To give you an idea of the kind of approaches currently being developed, I have included below a small sample of the types of therapies and tools which have proved to be the most effective in providing this type of psychological support. The examples used here are based on scientific studies and research.

Cognitive behavioural therapy

This type of psychological counselling enables patients to relate their thoughts and emotions to substance consumption and teaches them to modify how they think and react to the typical signs of substance use.

The procedure for this kind of therapy normally begins with the patient identifying critical situations and subsequently breaking these down into smaller episodes to pinpoint exact moments and associated behavioural factors. Each of those specific moments are then analysed in terms of the emotions and thoughts which trigger the resulting actions, with an in-depth analysis of their origin. Strategies are then devised to avoid those situations arising.

For example, one such critical situation could be the presence of alcohol at a party with friends. The party itself could then be broken down into critical moments, such as when a friend offers you a drink or says "Come on, it's just this once". This is a critical moment, a situation likely to trigger many emotions and thoughts which may lead to a relapse. Cognitive behavioural therapy hones in on these emotions and thoughts and analyses the deep-seated reasons behind them and how to overcome them when they arise.

Motivational interviewing

This type of counselling is an approach through which patients are encouraged and motivated not to give up treatment but to continue with it. The most common procedure is to use techniques to highlight the advantages and benefits to be obtained, whilst simultaneously attempting to invoke self-motivation and conviction in patients. In other words, the end objective is for patients themselves to reach the conclusion that all this effort is really worthwhile. These interviews primarily consist of a series of questions designed to encourage patients to reflect on and discuss their situation.

It is important for this type of counselling not to be seen as a strategy to convince patients of something, and particularly to avoid confrontation and the sense of imposition. Failure to achieve this generally causes the opposite effect to the one desired.

Positive reinforcement

Research on this subject has provided considerable evidence that rewarding positive behaviour in some way may be beneficial in this type of treatment. Recognition for achievement, adapted to the interests and situation of the patient, may be an interesting initiative.

A supportive environment

In recent years, increasing relevance has been given to addiction treatment therapies in which attention is not exclusively focused on the patient but also on the people around them, mainly their relatives and friends, who are often also seriously affected by the problem. In these new approaches, these people are involved from the outset and in all stages of treatment to ensure they take active part in the therapies discussed above. Their role is primarily to give support, to encourage, to "be there" when the patient needs them and to give them love and affection.

In this respect, one of the most used methodologies is known as CRAFT (*Community Reinforcement Approach and Family Training*). This approach has led to a significant increase in the prospects of recovery and would, therefore, seem to be providing promising results. For obvious reasons, this type of therapy is particularly useful and necessary in cases of addiction to substances which have a serious effect on patients, severely altering their behaviour and frequently destroying relations with their family and all those around them.

Treating possible food addiction

Now that we've looked at how substance addiction is treated, I'm sure it will be of interest for you to correlate these types of treatment with possible food addiction. Though I am aware of the fact that the lack of research on this subject and its possible clinical application prevents any comment on this issue from being anything more than a mere hypothetical intellectual exercise, I shall, nevertheless, give you my ideas on the subject. And I encourage you to give it some thought as well.

To start with, in the case of foods, one of the symptoms provoking considerable controversy is the concept of withdrawal syndrome, especially as it overlaps with the "normal" hunger we feel for homeostatic reasons. So, we're confronted with a complicated and unresolved issue right from the start. In any case, if food-related withdrawal symptoms *really* exist, it's possible to say that their intensity and effects are, with exceptions, generally less extreme and of a less serious nature than those provoked by most other substances. Furthermore, if customisation of treatment is an important factor in dealing with drug addiction, then this is also likely to be the case with food addiction.

In this case, what approach could be followed to maintain abstinence? As you obviously can't stop eating altogether, attention would need to be focused on specific foods. The first thing would be to devise some kind of method for identifying the most "addictive" foods, those which people are most likely to eat excessively and uncontrollably and which trigger that sense of craving. Brain imaging technology such as fMRI may be of great use in this respect, as could structured and systematic analysis of the behaviour and emotions associated with eating those foods. In this sense, the most useful resource is probably the Yale Food Addiction Scale (YFAS) that we looked at in the second part of this book. This scale enables us to rate the degree of addiction an individual may have (remember, the diagnosis starts to be considered as positive if the patient in question responds positively to at least three of the nine symptoms in the course of a month or more frequently, whilst at the same time feeling considerable distress) and to analyse which foods are associated with those symptoms. The "Palatable Eating Motives Scale" questionnaire, used to identify the emotional reasons behind eating, may also be of use.

Let's take another look at the main suspects likely, according to studies, to provoke a possible addiction:

- Chocolate, sweets, pastries, biscuits, ice-cream and desserts.

- Intensely-flavoured and rapidly-absorbed snack foods (crisps, corn and potato snacks, crackers, etc.).

- Fast food (pizza, pre-cooked and battered foods, etc.)

- Pasta, bread and rice.

Depending on how many of these foods are involved and the effects they provoke, different decisions could be taken within the fifth guideline (*Rewire your reward circuit*) discussed in the previous section: for example, total abstinence, as is normally the case with substance addiction (this could be applied in the most serious cases and/or if the "guilty" foodstuffs are few in number), or a controlled and programmed (daily, weekly, etc.) intake in small doses to see if this can be maintained.

Another interesting option could be to consider substituting the most craved-for foods (those which provoke a reaction similar to withdrawal symptoms and a harrowing feeling of distress) for others which bring about a sufficiently high sense of satisfaction without provoking any negative symptoms, disorders or distress. Examples of this could be to replace the slice of cake you normally eat for dessert with a natural yogurt with nuts and a sweetener, to substitute the bun you eat for breakfast for a vegetable and egg omelette or to do away with those after-dinner sweets and eat a little black chocolate (with a high percentage of cocoa and low sugar content) instead. Try to ensure that these alternatives are satisfying enough (though not excessively so) for them to be effective as replacement foods.

Similarly, another recommendation would be to follow the advice set out in the fifth guideline regarding "reprogramming" your brain. Shape a lifestyle for yourself in which healthy eating takes pride of place in your brain and healthy foods are once again perceived as tasty and appetising: learn as much as possible about those foods, take particular interest in selecting and shopping for them, cook them imaginatively and caringly and enjoy eating them. As mentioned in the 10-point-plan itself, studies would suggest that doing this can help rewire your reward circuit in favour of these foods and mitigate the expectations triggered by dopaminergic neurons in relation to less recommendable foods.

To date, little rigorous research has been conducted on the usefulness of cognitive behavioural therapy in treating obesity. Going back to the Palatable Eating Motives Scale, the twenty reasons for eating listed in the questionnaire are related to emotional and social factors, so this type of therapy is quite likely to be useful when attempting to identify those situations which spark the need in us to seek out undesirable foods, to break those situations down into more specific and detailed moments and to analyse the thoughts and emotions those same situations trigger in us. Cognitive behavioural therapy would undoubtedly help to define strategies to address these situations in a planned and structured way.

Let's once again use the example of being at a party with friends as a potentially conflictive situation. The most critical moments are likely to be when someone asks you "Are you on a diet?", or when someone encourages you to eat something you've decided not to by saying "Come on, it's just this once", or perhaps when the host brings out a dessert full of things you have decided not to eat but there's no other dessert on offer. An in-depth analysis of those moments, detailing the emotions and thoughts triggered by them in your head, understanding the reasons behind those thoughts and anticipating your possible reactions and specific behaviour in each case will all help to determine different ways of facing up to those moments without losing control.

As regards motivational interviewing, I believe the inclusion of motivational variables may be beneficial to this approach as a whole. Indeed, a self-analysis approach, led by a professional in this methodology, involving time for positive reflection, consolidating and reaffirming ideas and plans and reminding the patient of the crucial arguments underpinning the situation is usually highly effective. Furthermore, the use of positive reinforcement as a reward (or to reward oneself) for achievement has been seen to be useful in other contexts and could be a beneficial and pleasant way to go about things.

Support from family and friends would also be of critical importance in the potential treatment of food addiction. A supportive environment is an extremely powerful tool in helping to convince patients, especially children, who not only need to be motivated but educated in the matter. However, though the other therapies under discussion here *are* currently sometimes used in treating obesity, to actively engage family and friends in such treatment is a much more difficult proposition: due to the dominant stigma surrounding this issue, obesity is still perceived and considered as a fundamentally "personal" battle.

And that really just about completes what I have to say on the issue for the moment. I personally think that a lot can be learnt from addiction treatment: if things are taken forward with due care and attention, I believe new therapies customised to the reality of obesity can be developed which may be useful in addressing certain recovery processes, especially the most difficult ones.

In view of the level of interest in this issue, I trust that science will continue to advance in this field.

REFERENCES

Inside Rehab: The Surprising Truth About Addiction Treatment—and How to Get Help That Works (Fletcher, 2013)

Addiction Medicine: Closing the Gap between Science and Practice (2012)

Psychosocial Interventions for Mental and Substance Use Disorders: A Framework for Establishing Evidence-Based Standards (IOM, 2015)

Treating addiction-a guide for professionals (Miller et al, 2011)

Efficacy and safety of pharmacological interventions for the treatment of the Alcohol Withdrawal Syndrome (Amato et al, 2011)

Efficacy of interventions to combat tobacco addiction: Cochrane update of 2012 reviews (Hartmann-Boyce et al, 2013)

Cochrane systematic reviews in the field of addiction: past and future (Amato et al, 2013)

Levels of evidence in drug therapy for alcohol use disorders and illicit drug use (Burucker et al, 2012)

The effectiveness of psychosocial modalities in the treatment of alcohol problems in adults: a review of the evidence (Martin et al, 2012)

Behavioral counseling after screening for alcohol misuse in primary care: a systematic review and meta-analysis for the U.S. Preventive Services Task Force (Jonas et al, 2012)

A systematic review of evidence for psychological treatments in eating disorders: 2005-2012 (Hay, 2013)

What are the most effective techniques in changing obese individuals' physical activity self-efficacy and behaviour: a systematic review and meta-analysis (Olander et al, 2013)

Effective behaviour change techniques in the prevention and management of childhood obesity (Martin et al, 2013)

Motivational interviewing strategies and techniques: rationals and examples (Sobell et al, 2008)

Long-term effect of motivational interviewing on dietary intake and weight loss in Iranian obese/overweight women (Saffari et al, 2014)

Effectiveness of a motivational interviewing intervention on weight loss, physical activity and cardiovascular disease risk factors: a randomised controlled trial with a 12-month post-intervention follow-up (Hardcastle et al, 2013)

Motivational Interviewing in Childhood Obesity Treatment (2015)

A systematic review of motivational interviewing for weight loss among adults in primary care (2015)

Behavioral therapy for management of obesity (Jacob et al, 2012)

Psychological and behavioural factors associated with long-term weight maintenance after a multidisciplinary treatment of uncomplicated obesity (Buscemi et al, 2013)

3.3. A MOTIVATED BRAIN

The *National Weight Control Registry* (NWCR), set up to investigate long-term weight loss, was founded in 1994 by two North-American scientists. The main objective of the NWCR is to compile data on people who have lost at least 13.6 kg (30 lbs) of weight and kept it off for at least one year. The NWCR currently holds information on around 10,000 volunteers, and this information has been instrumental in conducting several other research studies.

The latest NWCR research findings, and particularly those related to people who have kept their weight off for longer periods of time (for example, for over 10 years), show a wide variety of methods are used to do so. However, practically all of these cases have one thing in common: considerable changes in lifestyle habits, especially those considered to be unhealthy. The conclusion to be drawn from these findings is *not* that the most important thing is to change, as "change for change's sake" makes little sense. What these findings really reveal is that the phenomenon of obesity is truly complex, and that it is very often necessary to change many things to win the battle against it.

Lessons learnt from addiction therapy processes may also be of help in fully appreciating the relevance of certain factors which are not always duly taken into account, especially those related to the psycho-social environment, emotions and psychology. If many changes need to be made to different habits and behaviour forms which are frequently and closely linked to a lifestyle centred on a particular substance, then the multidisciplinary support of professionals with expertise in these areas may be of great benefit in many cases. These experts will be in a position to provide help and advice on the complex process of undertaking changes which are often tantamount to rebuilding your life.

In any case, if this process of personal transformation is to have a minimal chance of succeeding, there is one ingredient in the mix which is absolutely essential: motivation. As we have seen before, the power of motivation is so strong that it enables many people to free themselves from complicated addictions just through their own efforts. The truth is that in this case, turning desire into reality is not a question of willpower, as stigma and prejudice would have us believe, but of motivation, and they are two very different things.

The scientific community has yet to give particular importance to motivation as a significant factor in losing weight. Attempts have been made by some experts to discuss this issue in greater detail but the truth is that researchers are not particularly motivated (if you will forgive the repetition) by the idea of including this concept in studies on obesity. Furthermore, when lists are drawn up on the key factors to take into account when managing health intervention plans and policies, motivation does not normally figure amongst them. Generally speaking, despite constant references to the need for changes in behaviour and habits, research studies on the mental conditions (motivation, for example) required to face up to and actually make those changes are, by and large, conspicuous by their absence.

Motivation is one of those holy grails that self-help books sell (and resell) continuously. The amount of interest in this issue should come as no surprise: after all, at some time in our lives we've all felt the need or desire to influence someone, to persuade someone to do something, to change something he or she is doing or to pursue a specific goal. I'm sure it's not too difficult for you to remember a situation in which you would have liked to know how to motivate your partner, or your children, or your colleagues at work, better. Or even yourself.

When we think about motivation we normally associate it with the idea of motivating someone. What comes to mind almost automatically are images of those preachers and conference speakers booming out their inspirational lines, or those captains and leaders of sports teams bringing the team together as one and getting the most out of each individual. However, this type of motivation has little value for us and is of no great interest in this case as it tends to be both volatile and extrinsic, i.e. difficult to sustain and driven by some kind of external "carrot on a stick" bait, incentive or reward. What's more, the effect of this type of motivation can normally be compared to that of an energy bar: a rush of excitement which quickly fades away to nothing.

In real day-to-day life, the most useful and enduring type of motivation is that which we develop ourselves, which comes from inside us. I'm referring to the motivation that drives us to do things "because I want to", not because "I've been encouraged to". Experts call this *intrinsic motivation*. This type of motivation does not involve carrots on sticks, or rewards, or brainwashing, and the only way it can be generated is by creating the right environment and context for it to come about and flourish on its own.

These conditions for motivation to flourish have long been well defined by sociologists and psychologists. However, this does not mean they are easy to achieve. One branch of psychology which has addressed and researched into the practical application of motivation with considerable success has been organisational psychology, where efforts are focused on identifying (and attempting to transform) human behaviour in the workplace. The thinking behind this is simple and clear: a motivated workforce generates greater value, both for the organisation and its customers, and enables the company to make more money. Companies and employers have long been aware of the fact that engaged and motivated people are more productive, more creative, more committed and produce better results. And therefore generate greater profits.

As a result, many writers have contributed a wide range of knowledge and different perspectives on this subject of human motivation in the business environment in recent decades. The books and specialised magazines published on the subject are almost too numerous to mention, though the fact that some of the authors are little more than peddlers of pseudoscience, opportunists and miracle sellers makes it necessary to separate the wheat from the chaff. Fortunately, after delving through these options for us, experts are of the opinion that the most interesting propositions are focused on and around the *self-determination theory*, an approach originally developed in the 1970s and centred on strengthening a person's autonomy, reducing external control and increasing decision-making options and capacity. A sizeable portfolio of studies and research, together with many real-life effective applications in fields such as education and job-seeking, have endorsed the usefulness of this theory.

Though definitions and approaches vary from one author to the next (depending on their need to "sell" new or supposedly revolutionary theories), the essential factors of intrinsic motivation can be boiled down to five key areas:

1. Minimising demotivating factors

2. Achieving autonomy

3. Seeking excellence

4. Relatedness

5. Being driven by a purpose

Let's look at these ideas one by one.

1. Minimise demotivating factors

Though it may seem an obvious and even redundant thing to say, it is important to have previously removed demotivating factors to be in a position of motivation. Eliminating those factors is no guarantee of achieving motivation, but their mere presence is an obstacle which is highly likely to prevent you from achieving it. In other words, confronting those *toxic elements* can be considered as a matter of hygiene, a cleansing action that needs to be performed to subsequently be able to address motivational strategies with a greater degree of success.

In the world of business such factors of hygiene, or hygienic factors, are normally considered to be things like salary, organisation and facilities, to name but three. All these issues are important - due care needs to be taken with them if people are not to feel dissatisfied – but experts have repeatedly shown that earning a lot of money or working in luxury facilities are not motivating factors in themselves. In other words, it's important and necessary to ensure these factors are of a sufficiently high standard, but this is not enough. They are mere preventive, or hygienic, measures.

Demotivating factors are also commonplace and easily recognisable in habit-changing processes focused on leading a healthier life. In fact, we have already spoken about them in previous chapters of this book when discussing some of the problematic situations associated with an obesogenic environment. Though each individual should identify their own personal demotivating factors and pinpoint those particular situations (frequently related to stress or emotional tension) most likely to sabotage their best intentions, a short indicative list is shown below.

- Habits which unsettle your metabolism (lack of sleep, sedentary lifestyle, lack of sunlight, overmedication, smoking, alcohol consumption, etc.)

- Situations of stress which may trigger emotional and compulsive eating (pressure at work, a lack of time, money problems, tension in personal relations, etc.)

- Access to unhealthy foods (lavish celebrations, supermarket shopping, storing unhealthy [or too much] food in the pantry, bad influences when eating, etc.)

- An unsatisfying diet (hunger, unpalatable food, eating hurriedly, etc.)

Though there is obviously no magic formula to solve the problems arising from each of these situations, it would be a good idea to sit down and think about each one of them and to identify the strategies you could follow to avoid them, minimise their occurrence or reshape them. If not, you may well find them troublesome. In any case, what's important is not to attach obsessive importance to them, not to overdramatise them or to take up an excessively radical stance in relation to them: these things sometimes happen, and you need to accept that. What you *do* need to do is to work on reducing their presence and the effect they can have, managing them calmly and sensibly. In this respect, the 10-point-plan proposed in the section entitled "Fixing the Thermostat" may be a good place to start, so I would advise you to read it again, to draw up a list of your own most common demotivating factors and to begin thinking about how best to address each one of them.

There is, however, another harmful factor which may create barriers and hinder motivation. This factor is particularly powerful as it stems from the brain itself, from the very same essence from which motivation should develop. I'm referring to negative beliefs, to those preconceptions and ideas we harbour and are deeply convinced of, normally because of some previous unsatisfactory experiences we may have had and interpreted as failures.

Negative beliefs in relation to losing weight can be summed up in three types of thoughts:

1. "Nothing works"

2. "I don't have enough willpower"

3. "I don't know enough"

These deep-rooted thoughts feed off our constant and unconscious struggle against cognitive dissonance. Such negative thoughts are very useful and convenient for us when we need to justify why we couldn't do something in the past: consequently, when faced with new ideas and possibilities, these thoughts fight tooth and nail to reject them. At the end of the day, they have a paralysing effect, impeding us from being objective and pressing us to reject most new proposals.

The third of these three negative beliefs is related to knowledge and competence but we'll look at that a little later when we address the issues of autonomy and excellence. What's important here to understand is that the other two, general scepticism and the sense of a lack of willpower, can only be combated in one way: by fully internalising the complexity of the problem of obesity, accepting that there are many other factors involved apart from personal responsibility and trusting in our ability, and in that of experts and scientists, to slowly come up with solutions. Everything we've been looking at and learning in this book may be helpful in this respect, as would further reading and study of specific literature (books and studies) on these negative thoughts and on specific dynamics and activities designed and piloted by specialist healthcare professionals, such as motivational interviews and group dynamics.

For example, approaches taken when attempting to dismantle demotivating thoughts of the "Nothing works" type could be rooted in the following:

- knowledge of what really has been proven not to work: the myths and historical errors regarding body weight and losing weight, and their origins;

- a catalogue of the trials and arguments that have been tested and followed (previous experiences, information, etc.) and which are now viewed with excessive scepticism. An analysis of the credibility of those experiences and what evidence would be required to reverse the situation;

- an analysis and knowledge of the specific and rigorous trials or actions which have been taken forward with a degree of success (albeit partial) through, for example, scientific studies and research; and

- looking into positive case-studies and testimonies with promising, though realistic, results, preferably from the immediate environment and which can be empathised with.

Similarly, the following ideas could be given in-depth consideration when attempting to refute the idea of not having enough willpower:

- an analysis of, and differentiation between, the concepts of *effort*, *priority*, *desire* and *motivation*, and of the variables which impact on them;

- a logical analysis and assessment of other common activities requiring a special effort (work, study, housework, etc.). Why do we do them?

- an analysis of things people enjoy doing which take up a lot of time and which, in theory, also require a special effort (family, hobbies, etc.). Why do we do them?

Whatever, a series of approaches for generating motivation are outlined below. Although these approaches are designed to progressively make demotivating thoughts subside, it is necessary to be aware of the existence of these thoughts, to accept that these assumed ideas have a considerable impact on our reasoning and to know what these thoughts are rooted in. If we can do this, we'll be in a position to work on and put forward initiatives and compile data and evidence to undermine them.

2. Achieving autonomy

On we go. If we can create an environment in which the previously mentioned demotivating factors are *reasonably* under control (reasonably... remember, perfection doesn't exist), we can then focus on creating the conditions in which intrinsic motivation can really be nurtured. Let's begin with autonomy. The fundamental axiom of the self-determination theory mentioned above is that *ideal* motivation is nothing more than getting people to feel the desire to do something on their own initiative. This can be achieved through two key approaches: autonomy and competence.

For people working in a company, autonomy is a question of being able to take your own decisions and, in a supporting role, to manage resources to be in a position to deliver the decision taken. Thus, it's necessary to ensure that those who so wish can be autonomous (in other words, that they can take decisions) and are provided with two types of resources: a thorough understanding of what's required to do their job (competence) and the resources required to act on their decisions. Criterion and resources. Mind and muscle. If a boss or manager wants his/her employees to feel autonomous, he/she must inspire trust and empower them by respecting the decisions they take, and support them by providing them with all the training, help and resources they may require at any time and in any area.

The same analogy can be drawn in the context of healthcare as in the world of business. For someone to feel sufficiently motivated to lead a healthy lifestyle and to be prepared to confront important changes in their life habits (with the idea of maintaining them long term), they must feel capable of designing their own best way to do this and of defining the steps required to do it. Healthcare professionals should, therefore, limit themselves to providing guidance in this respect, avoiding excessive control and patronising attitudes and reducing specific instructions to a minimum. Their main role should be to help the individual develop the desired sense of autonomy.

However, a good balance must be found: there is a thin line between autonomy and a sense of helplessness or abandonment. If the person in question feels abandoned, those demotivating thoughts we've just discussed will given a boost, and fear, paralysis and impotence will all gain ground.

In practice, how could these concepts be applied in the context of treating obesity and establishing a healthy lifestyle? How can someone be made to feel they have the competence and autonomy to achieve this goal? As I said before, the answer is essentially in the key idea that an individual will only feel competent and autonomous when they perceive they are in control of their initiatives and progress, are capable of understanding the problem and are able to define and roll out what needs to be done and how to do it.

If this is to be so, there are three things the individual in question requires a solid knowledge of: the real and primary reasons behind obesity, the basic principles for fighting against it and how to apply all of this, including the logic behind it, in practice. The first of these three issues has been the main focus and content of this book: a greater range of educational resources on this issue would be ideal. The second issue, the basic principles involved in combating obesity, can be directly addressed by applying the ten basic principles or guidelines discussed in the section entitled "Fixing the Thermostat". To remind you, these guidelines are once again listed below:

1. *Help your hypothalamus and digestive sensors to do their job well*

2. *Keep your glucose and insulin levels under control*

3. *Prevent leptin resistance and chronically high concentrations of this hormone*

4. *Avoid chronic or systemic inflammation*

5. *Rewire your reward circuit*

6. *Don't critically disrupt your circadian rhythms*

7. *Look after your microbiota and your microbiota will look after you*

8. *Be sceptical and critical about food marketing*

9. *Minimise stress*

10. *Keep active and do exercise*

With this list in mind, autonomy could be defined as the ability to fully understand what lies behind each of these ten principles.

The third issue, the ability to establish methodologies and apply them, would involve shaping the behavioural and lifestyle changes required to actually put all of these guidelines into practice. This is where expert and multidisciplinary support has a key role to play.

Make no mistake: to achieve all of this is by no means easy. The phenomenon of obesity is so complicated and the factors behind it so complex and misunderstood that, in terms of a strategy to fight against it, ignorance, a lack of control and not knowing where to start are all ideas that come to mind much more readily than that of autonomy. Just think, for example, of the huge amount of new food products available on the market, as diverse as they are mysterious from a health perspective. If it's so difficult for us to choose something as simple as the healthiest breakfast cereal, how are we going to be able to manage everything else that's involved?

Well, it can be done. Just like any other educational or learning process involving complex issues, it will require time and a rigorous approach backed up by solid evidence and expert opinion and the use of advanced educational techniques and approaches focused on promoting self-directed learning and decision making. For example, one possible approach cutting across all ten guidelines, and preferably piloted by a multidisciplinary group of professionals, could be to educate in, and encourage reflection on, the following:

- The identification and description of different types of foods and their components, especially in terms of their degree of processing, digestibility and metabolic and physiological impact (particularly on hormones such as insulin and leptin, on the microbiota and on inflammation). Specific literature, the use of databases, etc.

- Knowing how to handle, prepare and value fresh produce: ingredients, cooking processes, model recipes, tasting techniques, etc.

- Awareness of those external habits and factors which have a negative effect on the metabolic control system, and a knowledge of the mechanisms involved: sleep schedule, lack of exposure to sunlight, excessive indoor lighting and excessively warm environments, etc. Approaches to minimise these factors.

- Learning how to distinguish reliable and accurate sources of information on health from junk information and marketing. Provision and analysis of examples.

- Knowledge of techniques to control stress and anxiety and to organise one's time, task planning, defining priorities, etc. to help set aside time for leisure activities, the family, relaxation and meditation.

- Training in the principles and the latest types and trends of physical activity, exercise and sport, with detailed guidelines on how to do this exercise and its advantages and disadvantages. Trying out and practicing different types of sport to identify the one you find the most fun, challenging and satisfying.

Autonomy is obviously not something you can achieve from one day to the next. Far from being a one-off, isolated effort, we're talking of quite a long process, longer for some than for others, so progress will have to be checked regularly and the sense of autonomy and competence achieved assessed by personally consulting the individual in question. For example, this could be done by establishing a series of indicators which measure, or reflect, the individual's degree of intrinsic motivation in terms of interest, satisfaction and/or enjoyment, or by valuing and adjudging the sense of control or self-regulation the individual in question has acquired over his/her new habits. Adjustments to the training and learning actions could then be made accordingly on the basis of the findings.

As an example, below is a series of simple statements or items which could be included on a questionnaire to determine the degree of self-regulation an individual believes to have achieved in relation to the specific competence of *"design of a diet based on fresh foods"*. The individual under treatment could score each item on a scale of 1 to 7, with 1 expressing "I totally disagree" and 7 expressing "I totally agree".

1. I know how to select and combine fresh ingredients for the most appropriate type of cooked dish.

2. I know how to cook a stew and use the oven.

3. I know how to prepare a tasty dish using most of the vegetables available in the supermarket.

4. I know how to prepare a tasty dish using most varieties of poultry available in the supermarket.

5. I know how to prepare a tasty dish using most varieties of red meat available in the supermarket.

6. I know how to prepare a tasty dish using most varieties of fish available in the supermarket.

7. I know how to prepare a tasty and attractive dessert or afternoon snack using most varieties of fruit available in the supermarket.

Another type of questionnaire could be designed to measure indicators of motivation such as pleasure and satisfaction derived from the same habit or competence of following a diet based on fresh foods (using the same scoring scale). Items could include:

1. I eat fresh foods because I get told off if I don't.

2. I eat fresh foods because it's what I'm supposed to do.

3. I eat fresh foods because I'll feel guilty if I don't.

4. I eat fresh foods because it's important to eat healthily.

5. I eat fresh foods because I enjoy preparing them.

6. I eat fresh foods because I enjoy eating them.

In this case, a high score in the last items would indicate a greater degree of autonomy and of potential intrinsic motivation.

These are just simple examples provided for illustrative purposes. Many types of questionnaire have been drawn up by experts on the theory of self-determination (you'll have no problem finding them on the Internet) which could be used as the basis for drawing up new ones related to eating and other habits.

In short, on the path towards autonomy and competence, the role of the professional is not to provide an individual with overly specific and customised solutions but with a solid knowledge base with which to select and decide discerningly from among the options available. Furthermore, the professional should back this up with a wide range of methodological principles which enable the individual in question to actually put the possible lifestyle changes into practice. Only then will the professional be truly effective in helping the individual to feel genuinely motivated.

3. Seeking excellence

The next factor required to achieve motivation is, like autonomy, also related to knowledge and competence. However, in this case, we're not talking of knowing the basics, of knowing enough to reduce our sense of fear and to feel confident enough to take decisions. In this case, we're talking of something much more extraordinary, of something greater, of something called excellence.

Do you have a hobby? If you do, here's another question: what do you like about it? The answer to this second question normally takes a bit longer but if you think about it a little and are honest with yourself, you might come up with the answer "*because I'm good at it*" or "*because I'm quite expert at it*". Here's a third question: have you ever regretted stopping doing something you were particularly good at as a child? And one more question to finish: how do you feel when someone says to you "*you're really good at that!*". Great, I imagine.

Being particularly good at something is a very powerful motivator. We all want to feel a bit special and being recognised as being very good at something specific is something to treasure. The truth is that the phenomenon of excellence has been widely researched in psychology. The basic principles of excellence are relatively simple: being identified as being good at something drives us to do that activity more often. In doing so, we get better and better at it and enter into a vicious circle which, if maintained regularly over time, leads us on to a state in which our dominance of the activity in question becomes something intuitive, natural, spontaneous and relatively effortless.

Whatever, I can imagine what's going through your head reading this: Me? Excellent? Exceptional? I'm very normal. Well, study findings don't back you up so don't be so hard on yourself! I've personally seen that everyone I've met in my life has some kind of special gift, some kind of virtue, skill or ability they become particularly good at when they work on it a little. We're not talking about being a world-beater at something, just at succeeding at standing out somewhat in our own environment and among our own people.

The thing is that it's important to look for the opportunities to discover those things we can excel at. If we don't explore and try new things, the likelihood of finding something we excel at decrease significantly. In practice, the best way to seek out excellence is to follow the same recommendation as the one suggested for autonomy: learn. If you work hard at them, education and knowledge will help you develop all your skills and abilities, and it's highly likely that somewhere on that path, without even having planned it that way, you'll find you excel at something. If that happens, it won't be difficult for you to enter that vicious circle of excellence: you'll find yourself dedicating more time to it, a lot more time, you'll enjoy doing it and you'll get better and better at it.

At this point, it's important to make clear that although we are speaking here of education, one thing is to have a general and basic knowledge of something that helps us to take better decisions, but another is to find something that we really like and that we can really excel at. While both things are important, it's best to clearly distinguish between them. The first situation is related to autonomy, the second to excellence. Learning to cook is important, but earning the recognition of friends and family as an excellent cook of certain dishes (and even being encouraged by them to take part in a cookery competition) is something else. It's necessary to do some kind of exercise, but to be outstanding at one sport or another in your local area or among friends and to win competitions is exhilarating. To chat and share opinions with your friends is great but to write a blog and see that thousands of people are reading and following what you write is something to get hooked on.

In short, if you can face up to this profound process of change constructively and without becoming obsessed by it, it's quite possible you'll find something completely by chance that you particularly like and are good at. If this happens, it's important not to let this opportunity slip through your fingers: grab it with both hands, let your enthusiasm take you forward and enjoy it. Get into that vicious circle that drives you along the path to excellence, with the side effect of a considerable boost to your self-esteem. The net result will be a feeling of powerful motivation to continue with your change project.

4. Relatedness

As human beings, we are genetically programmed to interact and relate with others and to be sociable. Our physiology and metabolism are not that different from those of other living creatures, but our relatedness is infinitely more complex than that of other species. The cognitive superiority of our brain, the sophistication of language and the development of complex societies clearly reflect the sophisticated resources and mechanisms that nature has equipped us with to add a million and one nuances to our relations with our fellow human beings.

Feeling motivated triggers a strong will in us to develop interpersonal relations, which in turn makes us feel good. These relations may be of a close nature, such as with our emotional partner or close friends, or may be more superficial, such as with people we see more occasionally or the people from a group or some kind of association we are, or become, members of. Psychologists have shown that building up this kind of social network is beneficial in two ways: firstly, it provides support and understanding for the individual, and secondly, he/she feels more secure and protected. Though encouragement of this nature can also be obtained in several other ways, the first of the two benefits mentioned above is often essentially linked to personal relations and the second, to group or collective relations.

According to the theory of self-determination, perceiving that those around us are capable of covering both these emotional requirements is a key factor for motivation, and the activities themselves associated with creating and further developing our relations with these people is especially motivating in itself. In terms of the healthcare and lifestyle-changing perspective that concerns us here, the idea would be to introduce this variable of relatedness, in both the group and the more personal sense, into most of the processes of change and adoption of new habits. In this respect, new technologies provide a wide range of resources and possibilities to foster relatedness, but direct, face-to-face contact remains the most effective and natural for us.

Below are some examples of initiatives that could be taken to foster relatedness with others and thereby boost our intrinsic motivation in taking on new and healthy lifestyle habits.

- Group learning processes with people with similar need-to-know requirements.

- Joining some kind of group or association, e.g. a sports or mountain-walking club, a reading group, a gastronomy association, etc.

- Shopping for food with someone (a friend, your partner) who shares your concerns.

- Eating with groups of people with healthy eating habits and avoiding negative influences that go against healthy eating guidelines.

- Using on-line (forums, websites, blogs, social media, etc.) and specialist (recipe and exercise websites, amongst others) platforms to share ideas and experiences.

- The support of specialists (healthcare professionals, psychologists, coaches, etc.) trained in the required social skills (empathy, understanding, active listening, etc.) and in promoting autonomy.

Finally, and as mentioned above when discussing how to achieve autonomy, relational needs will also have to be checked regularly to measure the extent to which these activities are adding value and providing satisfaction for the individual in question.

5. Being driven by a purpose

The fifth and final factor involved in achieving genuine and lasting motivation, that of *purpose*, is rooted in the simplest yet most powerful and profound question of all: *why?* Or, put another way, *what's the reason for all of this and what's the purpose of it all*? Or, looking at the bigger picture, *what's my purpose in life*?

All this probably sounds too philosophical and general for you so allow me, if you will, to use another analogy. Most of us go about our lives like sailors, performing our duties and fulfilling our responsibilities whilst sailing in our boat. We get up in the morning, get dressed, have breakfast, clean the deck, lower the sails, row if there's no wind and repair whatever needs repairing. Maybe we socialise with our colleagues and, when the sun goes down and darkness falls, we rest. Day after day, month after month, year after year. If at some time we stopped to ask ourselves what we've done today, the answer would be "*sail*". This is logical... we're sailors. We go where the current takes us day to day, we get up, we work, we do what we have to do (sometimes that's interesting, sometimes not), we socialise with friends and family and at the end of the day, we rest. And the cycle goes on. We sail on.

But... where exactly is our boat going? What course are we sailing? Why are we sailing? People who take the decision to make some radical changes to their lives have often undergone some kind of unique experience that has forced them to ask themselves this question. Sometimes it's because they've taken some kind of enormous risk or have been in grave danger of dying: when this happens, they realise that their life as it is makes no sense or has no purpose. They are simply sailing, adrift, being carried along by the current.

As children, drifting rudderless may be understandable. Our brain lacks a future perspective and we are guided by our instincts to do what we like doing and what makes us feel good. However, as we get older, things slowly change. We start making plans about our future career, family and the lifestyle we want. In other words, we have a purpose or a goal. We design and shape our future, some of us in more detail and more ambitiously than others. We may not do this in a particularly considered and structured way but we decide on a course and destination for our particular boat and follow it for quite a few years. And when we have to take important decisions, this course and end destination play an important role in our thought process.

Paradoxically, this purpose tends to fade away with time. Maybe because the day-to-day problems and responsibilities of life increase as we get older and we have no time to think of the future... it's difficult enough to survive in the present! Or maybe because our long-term plans have been delivered or, conversely, have become impossible to achieve and we've given up on them. And that purpose we had when we were younger disappears, never to be replaced or updated with another.

In business, the most competitive companies use what's called a vision statement, or a statement of their end goal, as a guiding light. For them, it's essential to want to go somewhere, to want to *be something*, to want to feel something. Everything they do, every objective they set and every project they take forward makes a lot more sense in this context. And as people, we're really no different. Those people who really change and take the reins of their life are those with a defined purpose, a vision of the future they want for themselves, and they follow the path towards it. Scientific studies have shown that those people are the happiest, most motivated and healthiest.

At this point, you may be asking yourself... *And if I don't succeed? And if I become obsessed with this idea? Will I feel unhappy and frustrated?*

Good questions. Don't confuse having a vision or purpose in life with obsessively pursuing a specific objective. Remember: in the words of Allen Saunders, an American journalist (though this quote is commonly attributed to John Lennon), *"life is what happens to us while we are making other plans"*.

An ambitious and challenging goal can give our life meaning but there are plenty of other things that can do the same. Essentially, this is a personal decision. There are many effective ways to start thinking about this issue but, on the evidence of the most extreme cases, perhaps the most effective (and starkest) of all is to realise that you'll soon be dead. Take some time to think seriously about this and take this reality onboard. After all, there is but one absolute truth: all of us, sooner or later, are going to die. Maybe you or I will be amongst those people who die sooner than expected. I don't want to appear callous by saying that but that's often the way it is, and there's no point conning ourselves: it's an unfortunate reality that there's more chance of this happening than of you winning the lottery.

OK. I completely understand if you feel uncomfortable reading this but before you decide to skip this part of the chapter, I'd simply ask you to try to put yourself in a situation in which you can believe it. Imagine, for example, you've been told you only have a few days to live. Think about that situation and everything it would mean and then, ask yourself this question: what would you regret and what would you like to do with your life if your days on this earth were numbered?

Information is also available on the answers to these questions. Bronnie Ware, an Australian writer who has worked with people in palliative care, identified and compiled information on the five biggest regrets of those people conscious of the fact that they were soon going to die. The answers were quite consistent. The two biggest regrets were *"not living the life I wanted to"* and *"working too much"*.

Here's a direct question for you: Would you like this to happen to you? Wouldn't you like to take greater control of your life and do things that satisfy you, apart from the things you have to do out of obligation?

Whatever, enough of this: let's return to the optimistic tone of the book. These ideas are in no way intended to seem morbid or pessimistic: when we set ourselves an end goal, it's best to do what's necessary to achieve it in a constructive, positive and enthusiastic way, and if that same goal makes our day-to-day life make more sense, we won't only feel motivated but satisfied and happy.

The 12 Steps treatment methodology commonly used by Alcoholics Anonymous (AA) was discussed in a previous section of this book. This methodology looks to achieve motivation through spirituality, by putting one's faith in a superior being, an all-powerful God that gives meaning to everything and provides the strength required to do whatever is necessary. This religious approach is something we are used to: we've lived with it for centuries and it's been used by millions of people to give meaning to their lives, especially those who have had to suffer considerable hardship and sorrow. However, it goes without saying that it's certainly not the only way to achieve motivation.

Your purpose or vision should be defined on the basis of the answers you give to a series of key questions. These are: 1) Realistically speaking, what would you like to achieve in your life? 2) What (and who) really makes you happy? 3) What do really enjoy doing and with whom? 4) What are your best memories? Who were you with? 5) What do you not want to regret when you look back on your life?

As you can see, although the pursuit of happiness is a key element when looking to draw up or define a vision or purpose, it's likely to prove less complicated than you imagine, at least from a neurological perspective. Scientists have observed that the more individual moments of happiness we live, the greater our general sense of happiness, and on this basis, research has been conducted to identify, characterise and analyse exactly what those moments are. One case in point is the study published on the findings of research to determine a mathematical model capable of predicting happiness. To do so, experts used Functional Magnetic Resonance Imaging (fMRI) to observe the brain activity of a group of people being subjected to different situations and simulations in order to identify the ones that made them feel happy. On the basis of the resultant data, they were able to draw up a mathematical formula capable of predicting the degree of happiness of many people with surprising accuracy.

$$\text{Happiness}\left(t\right) = w_0 + w_1 \sum_{j=1}^{t} \gamma^{t-j} CR_j + w_2 \sum_{j=1}^{t} \gamma^{t-j} EV_j + w_3 \sum_{j=1}^{t} \gamma^{t-j} RPE_j,$$

What this collection of letters and symbols tells us is that happiness not only depends on the number of individual moments of happiness and how recently they have been lived, but also on something else of fundamental importance: the difference between the reward received and the expectations we had of the situation in question.

In practice, what this would appear to mean is that we feel happier when reality exceeds our expectations. It therefore follows that it's a good idea to create reasonable and realistic expectations which are, at the same time, challenging, with mini objectives and goals, mini "victories" on a day-to-day basis, doing things for a reason. This will trigger our neurons into secreting dopamine every time we achieve something. Yes, that's correct: dopamine, that same neurotransmitter that drives us to seek out food and to take action, that motivates us and sets us on course to achieve an objective.

So, what exactly is the link between our plan to improve our health and to fight against obesity and all these ideas on purpose and motivation? I think it's quite obvious. If you want to lose weight to wear trousers which are two sizes smaller, or to look good on the beach, or to feel happier with yourself when you look in the mirror, or to feel a bit more attractive for your partner, then this type of objective may not prove sufficiently motivating for you to change many of your lifestyle habits and actually achieve your objective. On the other hand, if what you're looking for is a satisfactory life, a strong and healthy body with the energy and will to attempt to turn your dreams into reality and to take forward your different plans and ideas, and to share the enjoyment of this with your family and friends for many years to come, then that's a whole different story. And so is motivation. Because if this is the case, instead of seeing your diet as having to go without certain foods, you'll see it as choosing the food of greatest value for your body. And rather than seeing a workout in the gym as a chore, you'll see it as preparing your new body for your new life.

Create your purpose, your vision, your end goal, and give your life meaning by making weight loss an integral part of it! That's the key message of this fifth and final factor.

Where do I start?

There is, unfortunately, no universal method or formula for starting work on these factors of motivation, or at least, not to my knowledge. As all individuals and their situation and circumstances are different, you'll have to draw up your own plan on the basis of your particular concerns, priorities and preferences. The order in which I have presented them here may be the start-up sequence for each one of them, but the pace at which they are taken forward and the degree to which each one is applicable and relevant to any given individual is something each individual must decide.

For obvious and logical reasons, it's a good idea to first address the hygiene factors, as their mere existence may quickly thwart any promising attempts to achieve intrinsic motivation. Though it's likely to be impossible to eliminate them completely, it's important to get rid of the major demotivating factors, those most capable of sabotaging our self-control, and to minimise the others as much as possible.

After that, I think it's a good idea to start with autonomy. As this is essentially a question of education and learning, this is the factor that usually takes the longest to achieve. What's more, and as mentioned before, the process of becoming autonomous means training ourselves and learning, in the course of which we are likely to find our niche, that activity at which we excel.

Relatedness can be worked on at the same time as the previous factors. This factor is not absolutely essential for your success but the more you can develop and further your relations with those around you, the quicker you'll be in a position to consolidate your motivation.

And as for your guiding purpose, your vision, your end goal... well, start thinking about now! Slowly, but surely. Without deadlines, but with a clear commitment. If you do things this way, and if you are consistent and persevere, then one day, almost without realising it, that purpose will appear in front of you, bright and clear, showing you the path to follow.

REFERENCES

Weight-loss maintenance for 10 years in the National Weight Control Registry (Thomas y otros, 2014)

Effective behavior change techniques in the prevention and management of childhood obesity (Martin et al, 2013)

The Obesogenic Household: Factors Influencing Dietary Gatekeeper Satisfaction with Family Diet (2015)

One More Time, How Do You Motivate Employees? (Herzberg, 1968)

Toward a Psychology of Being (Maslow, 1968)

Why Do People Fail to Adopt Environmental Protective Behaviors? Toward a Taxonomy of Environmental Amotivation (1999)

Self-Determination Theory and the Facilitation of Intrinsic Motivation, Social Development, and Well-Being (2000)

Self-regulation and the problem of human autonomy: does psychology need choice, self-determination, and will? (2006)

Facilitating health behaviour change and its maintenance: Interventions based on Self-Determination Theory (2008)

Motivation, self-determination, and long-term weight control (2012)

Motivational dynamics of eating regulation: a self-determination theory perspective (2012)

Using self-determination theory to promote physical activity and weight control: a randomized controlled trial in women (2010)

Self-Determination Theory as a Fundamental Theory of Close Relationships (2008)

Drive: The Surprising Truth About What Motivates Us (Pink, 2009)

Why Motivating People Doesn't Work . . . and What Does: The New Science of Leading, Energizing, and Engaging (Fowler, 2014)

The top five regrets of the dying (Ware, 2012)

On the relation between meaning in life and psychological well-being (Zika et al, 1992)

Meaning in life: an important factor for the psychological well-being of chronically ill patients? (Dezutter et al, 2013)

Purpose in life and use of preventive health care services (Kim et al, 2014)

What makes a life good? (King et al, 1998)

Theory-based psychosocial factors that discriminate between weight-loss success and failure over 6 months in women with morbid obesity receiving behavioral treatments (Annesi et al, 2014)

A computational and neural model of momentary subjective well-being (Rutledge et al, 2014

3.4. FOR THE POWERS THAT BE

So far in this book, every recommendation or piece of advice offered has been directed towards you, the reader, as an individual with an interest in the issue of obesity and/or someone who may be affected by it. However, the reality is that the problem of obesity goes far beyond the individual. As I have said on several occasions in this book, the trend in obesity in all so-called developed countries throughout the world is steadily increasing. In those same countries, the quality of life of the people suffering from obesity is progressively deteriorating and medical expenditure has soared uncontrollably, thereby jeopardising the availability of funds for other healthcare requirements. Most of these countries have launched a series of campaigns and actions designed to put a stop to this epidemic, none of which have had any significant success. In fact, the best that's been achieved has been to merely slow the process down.

Instead of these half-hearted attempts, what governments and experts need to do is to tackle the issue of obesity head-on and in all its magnitude. Some estimates have put the negative effects of obesity on the inhabitants of this planet on a par with smoking and armed conflicts. However, what studies and trials unequivocally confirm is that combating obesity is not a question of a lack of willpower, and that blaming the obese for their problem and sending out messages like "make an effort, it's your problem" have absolutely no effect whatsoever.

It is to be hoped that the recent consideration of obesity as a disease proves to be a first step in this direction. If this new approach is to be followed up coherently, I firmly believe that providing those affected with a series of recommendations and training on the issue will not be enough. Political thinking on the issue must also be overhauled to correct what has been seen not to work and to find new, more effective solutions. With such powerful interests and forces at stake, any attempts to combat such a complicated situation should not be left exclusively in the hands of the individuals affected as this will clearly be insufficient.

Consequently, and in line with this belief, eight guidelines addressed to politicians, healthcare administrators, finance managers and anyone else with decision-making powers in the field of public healthcare strategy, especially in relation to overweightness and obesity, are presented below. The idea behind this is simply to put forward some evidence-based general guidelines which should be further detailed by specialists and experts in the different areas at a later stage.

1. Create a body of sound, up-to-date and evidence-based scientific knowledge on obesity and foods and their effect on health.

As research on nutrition is of no interest for pharmaceutical companies, funding for it generally comes from the public sector. Though this has its advantages, one disadvantage is that funds are limited, especially in times of austerity and when public opinion gives priority to other issues. Another is inefficiency, a term often associated with public research due to the danger it runs of settling for a research environment in which the prevailing studies (observational) are the least clinically and scientifically valuable and which, furthermore, provide very similar and redundant results. All this in a scenario characterised by a shortage of better designed and valuable intervention studies from which to draw practical conclusions.

Consequently, those with responsibility in this area should promote and safeguard the availability of funds earmarked for research on these issues, and set up effective control mechanisms to ensure the quality and usefulness of this research work. Special effort should also be made to secure capable, cutting-edge and expert scientists to lead these projects.

2. Explore new evidence-based treatments.

The main focus of scientific research in this field should be to design and run trials on new and potentially effective treatments. Decades have been spent on approaches based on the simple theory of energy balance, repeating the same treatments of limiting the amount of high-calorie foods and trusting in the individual's personal responsibility to follow these guidelines. I think it's about time we admitted that this doesn't work, to stop banging our heads against the wall time and time again and to innovate by looking for new approaches.

The arrival on the scene of young and capable researchers may help to do away with old dogmas and open the door to new hypotheses on treatment and to learning from other specialities (for example, from other disciplines such as substance addiction).

3. Promote a multidisciplinary approach.

As has been made clear repeatedly throughout this book, obesity is a complex and multifaceted phenomenon attributable to multiple variables rooted in our modern lifestyle and requiring diverse scientific disciplines to approach and address it. Any research and development of new treatments should be handled by multidisciplinary teams of nutritionists, doctors, psychiatrists, neurologists, psychologists and endocrinologists, amongst others.

Together, these experts will be able to secure the knowledge and discover the approaches required to find solutions.

4. Educate in nutrition and health objectively and independently, allocating funds and resources proportional to the importance of the end objective.

It is totally unacceptable that, at the time of writing, food pyramids recommending foodstuffs produced with refined carbohydrates as the basis of a human diet can still be commonly found, when all available evidence points to that very idea being totally mistaken. Furthermore, it is totally incomprehensible how a considerable chunk of the medical profession continues to vilify fats and cholesterol as being the main culprits of cardiovascular disease. It is also outrageous how food companies are given a platform in schools – often under the guise of some kind of dubious association or foundation – to "educate" children on eating, when we all know that their real intention is to sell their products. And finally, it is disgraceful how obese people have been made to suffer the same kind of social stigma as TB and AIDS sufferers did in the past, even at the hands of healthcare professionals.

Education on health, food and obesity must be rigorous, evidence-based and provided by suitably qualified professionals. It must also be provided for children, ordinary citizens and healthcare personnel as so required. In this respect, it is important to be crystal clear about the fact that in this sense, "education" does not mean "spreading the word" or "communicating". We're not talking about producing some kind of powerful video documentary (which studies, furthermore, have shown to be potentially counterproductive), or of handing out some leaflets or giving half a dozen talks on the issue. Parallels should not be drawn with campaigns to reduce the number of road accidents, or on road safety or drug use prevention, as they are totally different from what we're dealing with here. Not only do these campaigns have a relatively low degree of success but they are also designed to influence some kind of relatively simple behaviour through a specific message; for example, *"limit your speed, limit the damage"*, or *"clunk click, every trip"*, or *"say no to drugs"*.

In contrast, obesity is neither a consequence of something that happens at any one specific moment, nor a phenomenon that can be prevented by avoiding any one particular type of behaviour. Despite what some people might think, it's not a simple question of energy balance, of eating less and doing more exercise. As we've seen throughout this book, obesity is the result of several factors accumulated over time and of very diverse origin. Not even the specific programmes devised by renowned experts worldwide have proved successful as reliable protocols for a long-term solution to the problem!

I'm sure that psychologists and educationalists would have no problem in explaining to any politician that education requires time, resources, perseverance and effort; in other words, that it goes far beyond what we've just been looking at. There are no short cuts when it comes to empowering and educating people in a healthy lifestyle, good eating habits and nutrition. It makes no sense for children to spend thousands of hours of their lives studying literature, history, mathematics and foreign languages when health, good lifestyle habits and nutrition are merely incidental in compulsory education.

5. Tax unhealthy products and subsidise the healthiest ones.

Whatever food manufacturers may say, some foods are healthier (in the sense that it's a good idea to eat them often) than others (those which it's advisable to eat minimally). If the general idea is to promote the first type of foods in detriment to the second type, then taxes need to be administered in line with these principles: in other words, less healthy foods need to be taxed and healthier foods, those which it's advisable to eat more of, need to be subsidised.

Such measures have already been seen to produce positive results. In some countries, for example, taxes on sugary drinks have been raised, thereby increasing the price, whilst the price of water has been reduced. In these cases, results after a mere few months show a considerable reduction in the consumption of the first type of drinks and an increase in water consumption.

6. Greater stringency in the regulation of food marketing

Knowing what you know you, allow me to ask you the same question as I did when we were speaking about hedonic eating: do you think it's reasonable to leave the food sector to its own devices in terms of self-regulation, responding exclusively to customer needs and expectations identified through their buying patterns?

I don't want to convey the idea that this sector is especially malignant because that would not be true. Large food companies generate wealth, create jobs and are no different to any other companies doing business in an economic model like the one we have. Nevertheless, I think it's clear to see that creating and selling products based almost exclusively on the tastes and preferences of customers and regulated solely by food safety standards is not enough to ensure healthy eating. For this very reason, regulations governing food marketing should be rigorously applied as a top priority and a foil against rampant, hyped-up and misleading publicity.

Such publicity is particularly dangerous in this field. Expenditure on marketing in the food sector in the United States is hundreds of times greater than what the government spends, so the battlefield clearly favours one side. I therefore believe that statements made by food manufacturers on the possible health benefits of eating their products should be severely curtailed, or even prohibited. The best option would probably be to exclusively allow official healthcare organisations to conduct this type of campaign, and food marketing aimed at children should, in any case, be prohibited.

Technical and legal provisions obviously need to be made available to ensure compliance with all these new guidelines, and the required control mechanisms need to be established or strengthened.

7. Promote emotional and psychological welfare

A healthy mind is required to bring about a healthy body. As you've seen in this book, there's a lot of scientific evidence behind the popular saying *"mens sana in corpore sano"*. A society in which many people are stressed, depressed or unhappy – in other words, a society in which mental health levels are at a minimum – is a seriously ill society.

These challenges should be met by drawing up and prioritising plans to address all these psychosocial needs: a comprehensive education programme, support for managing family and social relations, measures to ensure a proper work/life balance and the promotion of free time and leisure activities, amongst other initiatives.

8. Create healthy environments

The best preventive medicine against a multitude of chronic diseases, and especially for ensuring good neurological and cognitive health, is physical activity. Many modern cities have not been designed for the people who live in them but for cars and businesses. Towns and cities need to be remodelled and planned for people to be able to spend most of their time in a healthy environment, one in which they are not forced to put up with vehicle and factory pollution but are provided with wide-ranging and free sports facilities. An environment in which they can walk to work and to the local shops, go for a leisurely stroll and enjoy nearby green areas.

These issues are especially important when it comes to children. Studies have shown that children living in a natural environment with parks and grass and equipped with games and sports areas are more physically active. Conversely, in flat, paved areas, children tend not to run around so much and lead an increasingly sedentary lifestyle.

Additionally, user-friendly and practical pedestrian pathways and cycle lanes need to be built to make it easier for people to get around. More and bigger parks and green spaces need to be set up, playgrounds and sports facilities provided and attractive leisure options need to be made available for people and their families to spend their free time in a way which is more dynamic and active and less focused on consumption, shopping and mere commercial transaction.

REFERENCES

Global, regional, and national prevalence of overweight and obesity in children and adults during 1980—2013: a systematic analysis for the Global Burden of Disease Study 2013 (Ng et al, 2014)

Overcoming obesity: An initial economic analysis (McKinsey Global Institute, 2014)

Use of mass media campaigns to change health behavior (Wakefield et al, 2010)

Stand-alone mass media campaigns to increase physical activity: a Community Guide updated review (Brown et al, 2012)

Influence of price discounts and skill-building strategies on purchase and consumption of healthy food and beverages: outcomes of the Supermarket Healthy Eating for Life randomized controlled trial (2015)

Beverage purchases from stores in Mexico under the excise tax on sugar sweetened beverages: observational study (2016)

Assessing the potential effectiveness of food and beverage taxes and subsidies for improving public health: a systematic review of prices, demand and body weight outcomes (Powell et al, 2013)

Effects of a price increase on purchases of sugar sweetened beverages. Results from a randomized controlled trial (Waterlander et al, 2014)

Taxes on tobacco, alcohol and sugar sweetened beverages: Linkages and lessons learned (Blecher, 2015)

Access to excess: how do adolescents deal with unhealthy foods in their environment? (deVet et al, 2014)

The relationship between built environments and physical activity: a systematic review (Ferdinand et al, 2012)

A systematic review of built environment factors related to physical activity and obesity risk: implications for smart growth urban planning (Durand et al, 2012)

The Role of Built Environments in Physical Activity, Obesity, and CVD (Sallis et al, 2013)

Objectively measured differences in physical activity in five types of schoolyard area(Andersen et al, 2015

A HOPEFUL BRAIN

I hope this book has helped you to understand why obesity is such a complex and difficult issue to solve. Things are never easy when the brain is involved in issues like this. The book may also have given you another perspective on obesity, its origin and its social implications, as well as the possible solutions to this phenomenon which must necessarily go beyond and be more ambitious than the hackneyed standard of "eat less and do more exercise".

This book is the third in a series outlining the basic scientific concepts related to obesity and nutrition. As the author, my idea throughout has been to write about these issues in such a way as to make them interesting and entertaining for the general public. If you have no professional link to this subject and have simply read this book and/or the others out of interest, then I hope you've found them easy to read and useful. If, on the other hand, you are a specialist, a dietician, a psychiatrist, a neurologist or a psychologist, then it's likely that certain parts of the book may have fallen short for you, though I hope there have been others which have complemented what you already knew and aroused your interest to delve further and more rigorously into certain elements of the subject.

Above all, I hope this book has made you want to learn more, awakening your interest in science and your curiosity to find out more about nature and the wonderful world around us so full of surprises.

And finally, my thanks go to Gustavo Diaz and Unai Martínez, without whose contributions this book would not have been the same.

For further information on the writer, go to:

http://loquedicelacienciaparadelgazar.blogspot.com/
http://elcentinel.blogspot.com/

If you'd like to give me your opinion on the book or simply get in touch with me, e-mail me at:

elblogdecentinel@gmail.com

Below are the front covers of two other books I've written on food and health:

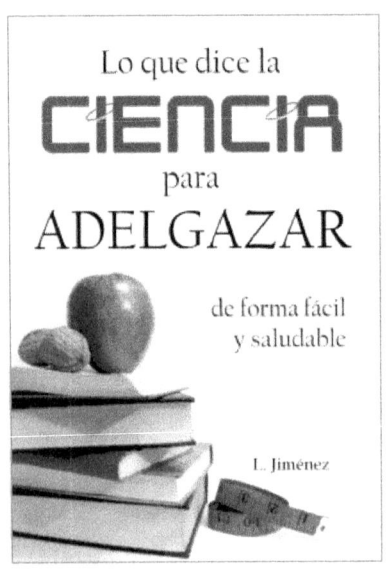

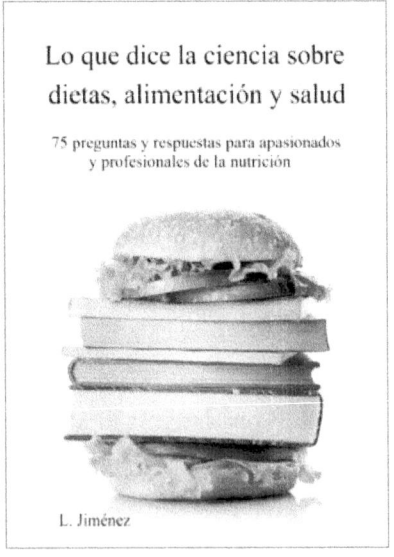

Many thanks for obtaining this book.

Luis Jiménez, May 2016

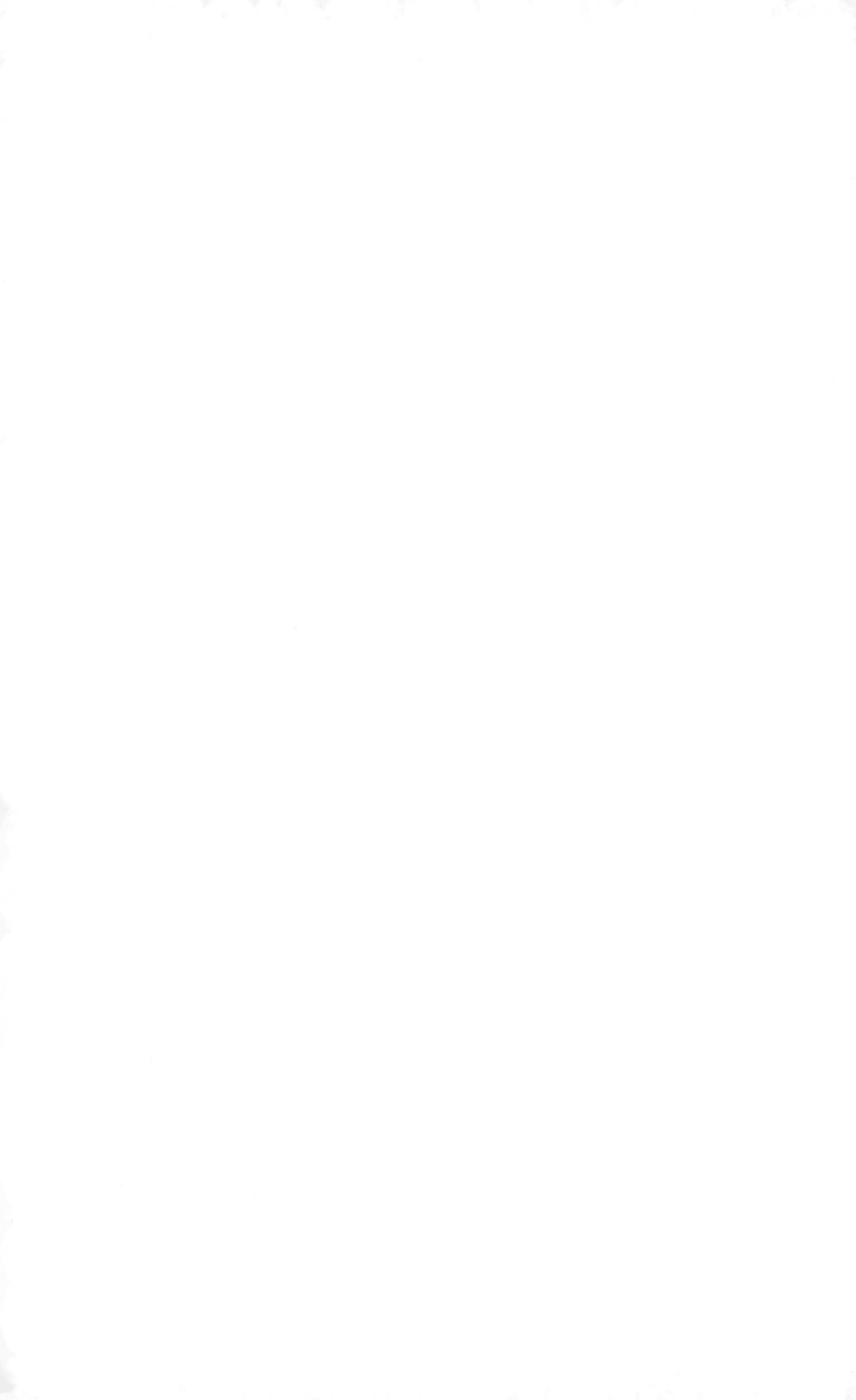

www.ingramcontent.com/pod-product-compliance
Lightning Source LLC
Chambersburg PA
CBHW070229190526
45169CB00001B/127